Bipolar Disorder: Treatment and Management

by

Trisha Suppes, MD, PhD
Paul E. Keck, Jr., MD

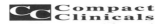

CC Compact Clinics

Medical Publishers   Kansas City, MO

This book is prepared and presented as a service to the medical community by arrangement with Compact Clinicals, which received funding support from AstraZeneca Pharmaceuticals LP. The information provided reflects the published literature as well as the knowledge, experience, and personal opinions of the authors, Trisha Suppes, MD, PhD, and Paul Keck, Jr. MD.

This book is not intended to replace or to be used as a substitute for the complete prescribing information prepared for each drug by its respective manufacturer. Because of possible variations in drug indications, in dosage information, in newly described toxicities, in drug/drug interactions, and in other items of importance, reference to such complete prescribing information is definitely recommended before any of the drugs discussed are used or prescribed.

Published by:
Compact Clinicals
7205 N. W. Waukomis
Kansas City, MO 64151
816-587-0044

Content Editing: Melanie Dean, PhD, Compact Clinicals
Copy Editing: In Credible English, Inc.®

Library of Congress Cataloging-in-Publication Data

Suppes, Trisha
Bipolar disorder : treatment and management / by Trisha Suppes, Paul E. Keck., Jr.
     p.   ; cm.
  Includes bibliographical references and index.
  ISBN 1-887537-26-0
  1. Manic-depressive illness. 2. Manic-depressive illness--Treatment.
  [DNLM: 1. Bipolar Disorder. 2. Bipolar Disorder--therapy. WM 207 S959b   2005] I. Keck, Paul E. II. Title.
RC516.S865 2005
616.89'506--dc22

                              2004027635

Printed in the United States of America
10 9 8 7 6 5 4 3 2 1

Table of Contents

Dedications

*To my mother and father,
with appreciation for their
unflagging support
(Trisha Suppes)*

*To Paul and Shirley,
for all their support
and sacrifices
(Paul Keck)*

Chapter 1: Introduction & History of Bipolar Disorder

Bipolar disorder, also known as manic-depressive illness, affects an individual's mood, behavior, and thinking. Symptoms vary as moods swing from the illness' manic phase (characterized by feelings of elation/euphoria, extreme optimism, inflated self-esteem, decreased need for sleep, engaging in risky activities, etc.) to the depressive phase (feelings of extreme guilt, sadness, hopelessness, anxiety, and, at times, suicidal thoughts). The symptoms of bipolar illness are severe and often life threatening; fortunately, bipolar disorder can be treated, and people with this illness can lead full and productive lives. Often an individual experiences periods of euthymia or "normal" mood between episodes of the two extremes.

Bipolar disorder typically develops in late adolescence or early adulthood; however, some people have their first symptoms during childhood, while others develop them late in life. Often unrecognized, people may suffer for years before obtaining an accurate diagnosis.

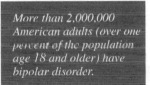

More than 2,000,000 American adults (over one percent of the population age 18 and older) have bipolar disorder.

Bipolar disorder affects both sexes equally, but women are about three times more likely to experience rapid cycling; that is, having four or more distinct periods of depression, hypomania, mixed states, or mania in a one-year period.

Both children and adolescents can develop bipolar disorder. Unlike many adults with the illness, whose episodes are more easily definable, children and young adolescents with bipolar disorder often experience chronic mood changes, including rapid mood swings between depression and mania many times within a day. Children with mania are more likely to be irritable and prone to destructive tantrums than to be overly happy and elated. Mixed symptoms also are common in youths with bipolar disorder. Older adolescents who develop the illness may have more classic, adult-type episodes and symptoms.

Bipolar disorder, however, can also appear for the first time in people over 40. The illness that develops in elderly people is less likely to be associated with a family history of the disorder and more likely to accompany medical and neurological problems than earlier-onset bipolar disorder.

Researchers are continuing to learn about the causes of bipolar disorder. Most scientists agree that there is no single cause; rather, many factors act together to produce the illness. Bipolar disorder appears to run in families, often affecting someone from every generation.

Mania: Hallmark Syndrome of Bipolar Disorder

What distinguishes bipolar disorder from unipolar depression is the presence of at least one manic episode characterized by:

- Increased energy, activity, and euphoria

- Increased restlessness, distractibility, irritability, and racing thoughts

- Decreased need for sleep

- Loss of rationality, poor judgment, and unrealistic beliefs in one's abilities

- Increased sexual urges and provocative behavior

- Risky behavior, poor judgment

- Drug abuse (particularly abuse of alcohol, marijuana, and sleeping medications)

Psychotic symptoms occur in at least 50 percent of manic episodes. In a delusional state, patients lose their perception of reality. For example, a person may believe they possess amazing strength and ability, are extremely wealthy, or are publicly desired. Auditory hallucinations are common and can be dangerous. The person may also develop paranoia.

Hypomania: A Mild-to-Moderate Level of Mania

Hypomanic individuals may feel great and even associate their symptoms with optimal functioning and enhanced productivity. Thus, even when family and friends learn to recognize the mood swings as possible bipolar disorder, the person may deny that anything is wrong. Without proper treatment, however, hypomania can lead to more severe mania or herald a period of ongoing mood instability.

Depression: The Other End of The Spectrum

After any manic episode, mild or severe, people with bipolar disorder may experience depression or a symptom-free phase. Eventually, in most untreated individuals, a depressive episode ensues. Symptoms of depression include a loss of interest or pleasure in activities once enjoyed (including sex), changes in appetite and weight, and decreased energy, concentration, and memory. Depression symptoms also include **increased** feelings of hopelessness, pessimism, guilt, worthlessness, anxiety, or helplessness, fatigue, irritability, or restlessness, chronic pain (not caused by physical illness or injury); and thoughts of death or suicide (including suicide attempts)

Many people present only with depressive symptoms, not recognizing manic or hypomanic periods. The differential diagnosis of unipolar (major depression only) from bipolar is critical for all patients presenting with depression.

Mixed Episodes: When Manic and Depressive Symptoms Occur Together

Symptoms of a mixed bipolar state often include agitation, trouble sleeping, significant change in appetite, psychosis, and suicidal thinking. A person may have a very sad, hopeless mood while at the same time feeling extremely energized and agitated.

Mixed episodes are often severe and impair daily functioning in social interactions, occupational activity, and intimate relationships. A mixed episode can last from one week to several months; generally followed by a depressive episode. Women are more prone to mixed episodes. In teenagers, mixed episodes occur most frequently among those who have experienced major depression, and for children this may be the primary presentation.

History of Bipolar Disorder and Its Classifications

Although nosology varies greatly, bipolar disorder has been recognized throughout recorded history. The modern concepts of bipolar disorder were formulated and refined during the 18th and 19th centuries. The mid-20th century saw the evolution of our understanding of bipolar disorder to a disorder with distinctive epidemiological, familial, and clinical characteristics that clearly differentiate it from unipolar depressive disorder.

Manic-depressive illness historically included both what is now termed bipolar illness and unipolar or major depressive illness. Individuals who experienced recurrent episodes of major depression were considered manic-depressive. DSM-III reflected the distinction of bipolar disorder from depression, dropping the older, more-inclusive term of manic-depressive illness utilized in DSM I and II.

This change in nosology reflected new thinking about affective illness and a new approach to identification and diagnosis of psychiatric illness that developed in the 1970s. During this period, a number of research centers presented the concept that diagnoses should be based on specific symptom and other

The timeline on the next page provides an "at-a-glance" perspective of this transition.

Table 1-1. Bipolar Disorder Timeline

Bipolar Disorder Timeline

Classical Period

300 BC - Hippocrates describes four humors and links to diseasevvv

200 AD - Aretaeus of Cappadocia suggests mania/depression symptoms are counterparts of same disease.

100 BC - Soranus of Ephesus describes mania as a remitting illness mixed with melancholia in some patients

19th & Early 20th Centuries

1851 - Jean-Pierre Falret publishes descriptions of "folie circulaire," a continuous cycle of depression, mania, and free intervals of varying duration.

1854 - Baillarger counters Falret's concept with "folie à double forme," which failed to acknowledge importance of symptom-free interval.

1877 - Hecker describes "partial mental disorder" as periodic changes of depression and exaltation, later given the name "cyclothymia."

1893 - Emil Kraepelin, establishes manic-depressive illness as a nosological entity recognizable as disease.

1900 - Wernicke asserts manic-depressive illness as a distinct entity rather than part of melancholia.

1911 - Kleist separates affective disorders into distinct unipolar and bipolar entities, maintaining that mania and melancholia are separate forms of monopolar psychoses occurring in the same person.

Mid to Late 20th Century

1957 - Leonhard subdivides phasic psychoses into "pure" and "polymorphous," with the latter containing manic-depressive illness.

1966 - Angst and Perris characterize bipolar illness as nosologically nonhomogeneous.

1976 - Dunner et. al. differentiates bipolar I from II.

1994 - Bipolar I and II dichotomy accepted for the first time in DSM-IV

1996 - Akiskal sees bipolar disorder as a spectrum, proposing bipolar III, higher disorders, subcategories for major subtypes.

Compiled from various sources[1-8]

DSM-IV(TR) terminology will be used throughout this manual.

validating criteria. The bipolar I and II dichotomy was accepted for the first time in the Diagnostic and Statistical Manual (DSM-IV) in 1994; however, hospitalization was not required for a diagnosis.

At present, the DSM-IV Text Revision (TR) includes the four subtypes shown in table 1-2.

Table 1-2. Bipolar Disorder Today [DSM-IV(TR)][9]

▲ Bipolar I Disorder
- ◆ Single Manic Episode
- ◆ Most Recent Episode Hypomanic
- ◆ Most Recent Episode Manic
- ◆ Most Recent Episode Mixed
- ◆ Most Recent Episode Depressed
- ◆ Most Recent Episode Unspecified

▲ Bipolar II Disorder
- ◆ Presence (or history) of one or more major depressive episodes (see chapter 3.)
- ◆ Presence (or history) of at least one hypomanic episode.
- ◆ There has never been a manic episode or a mixed episode (see chapter 3).

▲ Cyclothymic Disorder
- ◆ For at least 2 years, the presence of numerous periods with hypomanic symptoms (see chapter 3) and numerous periods with depressive symptoms that do not meet criteria for a major depressive episode.
- ◆ During the above 2-year period (1 year in children and adolescents), the patient has not been without the symptoms in Criterion A for more than 2 months at a time.

♦ No major depressive episode, manic episode, or mixed episode (see chapter 3) has been present during the first 2 years of the disturbance. Note: After the initial 2 years (1 year in children and adolescents) of cyclothymic disorder, there may be superimposed manic or mixed episodes (in which case both bipolar I disorder and cyclothymic disorder may be diagnosed) or major depressive episodes (in which case both bipolar II disorder and cyclothymic disorder may be diagnosed).

▲ Bipolar Disorder Not Otherwise Specified

Reprinted with permission of American Psychiatric Association, Diagnostic and Statistical Manual of Mental Disorders, Fourth Edition, Text Revision, Washington, D.C., American Psychiatric Association, 2000.

References

1. Angst J, Marneros A. Bipolarity from ancient to modern times: conception, birth and rebirth. *J Affect Disord.* 2001; 67(1-3):3-19.

2. Maj M. *Bipolar disorder.* New York: John Wiley & Sons; 2002.

3. Falret JP. Marche de la folie (suite). *Gaz Hop.* 1851; 24(18-19).

4. Dunner DL, Gershon ES, Goodwin FK. Heritable factors in the severity of affective illness. *Biol Psychiatry.* 1976; 11(1):31-42.

5. Akiskal HS. The prevalent clinical spectrum of bipolar disorders: beyond DSM-IV. *J Clin Psychopharmacol.* 1996; 16(2 Suppl 1):4S-14S.

6. Akiskal HS, Pinto O. The evolving bipolar spectrum. Prototypes I, II, III, and IV. *Psychiatr Clin North Am.* 1999; 22(3):517-34, vii.

7. Akiskal HS, Bourgeois ML, Angst J, Post R, Moller H, Hirschfeld R. Re-evaluating the prevalence of and diagnostic composition within the broad clinical spectrum of bipolar disorders. *J Affect Disord.* 2000; 59 Suppl 1:S5-S30.

8. Goodwin FK, Jamison KR. *Manic-Depressive Illness.* New York, NY: Oxford University Press; 1990.

9. American Psychiatric Association, American Psychiatric Association Task Force on DSM-IV. *Diagnostic and statistical manual of mental disorders: DSM-IV-TR.* Washington, DC: American Psychiatric Association; 2000.

Chapter 2: Epidemiology & Risk Factors of Bipolar Disorder

Epidemiologic studies indicate that bipolar disorder is a common and severe psychiatric illness. However, lifelong prevalence is possibly higher than published figures due to:

- Delay between onset of symptoms and diagnosis

- Under-reporting and under-recognition

- Stigma associated with mental illness

- Some cultural tendency to seek assistance from religious and other, non-medical support systems

Prevalence estimates of bipolar disorder range from 1.6 to 3.7 percent. Age of onset, ethnicity, and factors related to genetics, environment, and medical/psychological contributors can increase risk for the disorder.

Chapter 2 at a Glance

Epidemiology of Bipolar Disorder

This section addresses prevalence, gender, age of onset, and ethnic issues for adults with bipolar disorder.

Prevalence

It is difficult to determine the prevalence of bipolar disorder. This is because the diagnosis is not usually established at the time of initial presentation.[1] While mania is clearly a core feature of bipolar I disorder, hypomania (a core feature of bipolar II disorder) may be missed or dismissed as a personality characteristic.

Most patients with bipolar disorder seek help from primary care physicians when they are depressed; thus, a possible diagnosis of bipolar disorder may be overlooked.[2] Consequently, statistics on the incidence of bipolar disorder are retrospective. Frequency statistics generally rely on lifetime prevalence data.

In a population-based, cross-national epidemiologic survey of 38,000 patients from 10 countries, Weissman et. al. estimated that the lifetime prevalence of bipolar disorder (as compared to major depression) across countries was:[3]

- More consistent than major depression rates

- Undiagnosed on average for six years before patients seek help, typically for major depression, which can further extend the time from onset to bipolar diagnosis

- Consistent, reflecting the absence of cultural risk factors influencing epidemiology of major depression

Two major community surveys of the U.S. general population confirmed the findings of Weissman et. al.[4, 5] Additional data from the National Comorbidity Study estimated prevalence of 1.6 percent.[6]

The American Psychiatric Association suggests that these overall rates of bipolar disorder may be conservative.[7] Hirschfeld et. al. utilized the Mood Disorder Questionnaire (MDQ) — a sensitive but non-specific, validated screening tool for bipolar disorder — to determine the prevalence of bipolar I, II, and bipolar NOS disorders in the U.S. general population, finding 3.7 percent of the general population screened positive for a possible bipolar disorder.[8]

Gender

The overall incidence of bipolar disorder is approximately gender neutral. However, epidemiological studies indicate that bipolar II disorder, a condition in which depressive episodes predominate, may be somewhat more common in women.[9]

> *Since unipolar depression is so much more common in women, any man presenting with major depression should be evaluated for bipolar disorder as well.*

Age of Onset

Although bipolar disorder can present at almost any age, research indicates a peak period of onset in late adolescence (ages 15–19).[1, 10] Onset at the age of 30 years or older was less common; only 16 percent of subjects reported onset of symptoms during this time of their life.

Ethnic Issues

Although bipolar disorder appears to be no more prevalent among any one ethnic group than another, African Americans with schizoaffective disorders (including the bipolar subtype) are under-diagnosed in favor of schizophrenia or other non-affective psychoses. This is apparently due to an interpretative or diagnostic bias identified in the United States, the United Kingdom, and the Caribbean.[11, 12]

> *Consider bipolar disorder in all patients presenting with affective complaints, regardless of race.*

Risk Factors for Bipolar Disorder

A number of variables can influence an individual's risk of clinical manifestations and susceptibility to bipolar disorder.

While the disorder has a strong genetic component, it is probable that development of, and vulnerability to, the illness is also influenced by an interaction of genetic, environmental, perinatal, medical/physiological, and psychological factors.[2]

Genetics

Data from large numbers of family studies as well as adoption studies demonstrate a consistent relationship between family history and risk of bipolar disorder.[13, 14] In family studies, at least two-thirds of patients with bipolar disorder have a family history of affective illness.[14] The risk increases with the presence of major affective illness in parents. If one parent has a major affective disorder, the children have about a 20 to 25 percent risk of also being affected.[15] If both parents have an affective disorder, and one is bipolar, the children have a 50 to 75 percent risk of affective illness.[16]

Some of the strongest evidence for the genetic component of bipolar disorder comes from twin studies. Bertelsen et. al. studied a population of 11,288, same-sexed twin pairs born 1870–1920 in Denmark.[17] The study identified 126 probands from 110 pairs and reported concordance rates for bipolar disorder of 62 percent for monozygotic twins and 8 percent for dizygotic twins, resulting in an estimated 59 percent heritability of the disorder for twins.

The exact mode of bipolar disorder inheritance is unknown. Evidence points to susceptibility loci on multiple interacting genes.[18] The strongest evidence supports a role for genes on chromosomes 18p, 18q, and 21q.[19] However, methodological issues make it difficult to convincingly confirm the significance of these loci at this time, due to the fact that they are susceptibility genes, each of which has relatively little influence alone. The genes may either confer susceptibility in limited numbers of families, or sample sizes of various studies are too small to rule out associations by chance alone. Efforts are ongoing to identify and characterize specific susceptibility loci.

Medical/Physiological and Psychological Contributors

Many medical/physiological diseases/factors can precipitate or exacerbate bipolar disorder manifestations.

Perinatal Complications

There appears to be an association between perinatal complications and risk of mental illness. Several studies describe an association between schizophrenia and obstetrical complications (e.g., degree of parity, maternal bleeding, season of birth).[20, 21] However, the possible association is not as well studied in bipolar disorder.[2, 22]

Reproductive Cycle/Post-Partum Impacts

In women, bipolar disorder can be associated with events of the reproductive cycle and the post-partum state. Of women with bipolar disorder, it is reported that 66 percent may experience premenstrual or menstrual exacerbations of mood symptoms, and approximately 25 percent may experience premenstrual depression.[23] Ongoing, prospective studies are expected to provide more hard estimates of the clinical impact of monthly hormonal changes. During the post-partum period, women at risk for bipolar disorder face an increased risk of onset; similarly, those in remission face a greater risk of relapse.[24]

Thyroid Disease Impact

Some patients with thyroid disease may be at increased risk for bipolar disorder, perhaps because thyroid hormone has significant effects on brain metabolism and neural activation. For example, triiodothyronine (T3) may accelerate and augment antidepressant response to tricyclic antidepressants in patients with refractory unipolar depression.[25] Patients with bipolar disorder have been shown to have an increased incidence of antithyroid antibodies compared to controls.[26] In fact, the presence of significant titers of antithyroid antibodies is higher in bipolar patients than in those with other affective disorders.[27]

Cyclothymia

A risk factor for bipolar disorder, episodes characteristic of cyclothymia (fluctuating mood disturbance involving numerous periods of hypomanic and depressive symptoms) are common in patients with bipolar disorder. To determine the clinical course of cyclothymia, Akiskal et. al. found that the presence of cyclothymic manifestations should be considered indicative that a patient may eventually manifest classical symptoms of bipolar disorder.[28]

Environmental Contributors

Although genetics plays a strong role in the genesis of bipolar disorder, concordance rates less than 100 percent among monozygotic twins support the role of environmental factors as well as more complicated genetic penetrance patterns. It is reasonable to postulate that genetics plays a stronger role in those with early-onset disease.[2]

Studies of socioeconomic influence have been conflicting, alternately suggesting that bipolar disorder is more common in either those of higher or lower socioeconomic status.[1, 29]

Major life stressors can influence the course of illness. Stressful events can precipitate relapse.[30] Alternately, life events associated with positive goals can increase manic symptoms.[31] Changes in sleep-wake cycles that occur with sleep deprivation or international travel can also precipitate or exacerbate manic, hypomanic, or mixed episodes.[32]

References

1. Bebbington P, Ramana R. The epidemiology of bipolar affective disorder. *Soc Psychiatry Psychiatry Epidemiol.* 1995; 30(6): 279-92.

2. Rush AJ. Toward an understanding of bipolar disorder and its origin. *J Clin Psychiatry.* 2003; 64 Suppl 6:4-8; discussion 28.

3. Weissman MM, Bland RC, Canino GJ, Faravelli C, Greenwald S, Hwu HG, Joyce PR, Karam EG, Lee CK, Lellouch J, Lepine JP, Newman SC, Rubio-Stipec M, Wells JE, Wickramaratne PJ, Wittchen H, Yeh EK. Cross-national epidemiology of major depression and bipolar disorder. *JAMA.* 1996; 276(4):293-9.

4. Regier DA, Farmer ME, Rae DS, Locke BZ, Keith SJ, Judd LL, Goodwin FK. Comorbidity of mental disorders with alcohol and other drug abuse. Results from the Epidemiologic Catchment Area (ECA) Study. *JAMA.* 1990; 264(19):2511-8.

5. Regier DA, Myers JK, Kramer M, Robins LN, Blazer DG, Hough RL, Eaton WW, Locke BZ. The NIMH Epidemiologic Catchment Area program. Historical context, major objectives, and study population characteristics. *Arch Gen Psychiatry.* 1984; 41(10):934 41.

6. Kessler RC, McGonagle KA, Zhao S, Nelson CB, Hughes M, Eshleman S, Wittchen HU, Kendler KS. Lifetime and 12-month prevalence of DSM-III R psychiatric disorders in the United States. Results from the National Comorbidity Survey. *Arch Gen Psychiatry.* 1994; 51(1):8-19.

7. American Psychiatric Association: Practice guideline for the treatment of patients with bipolar disorder (revision). *Am J Psychiatry.* 2002; 159(4 Suppl):1-50.

8. Hirschfeld RM, Calabrese JR, Weissman MM, Reed M, Davies MA, Frye MA, Keck PE, Jr., Lewis L, McElroy SL, McNulty JP, Wagner KD. Screening for bipolar disorder in the community. *J Clin Psychiatry.* 2003; 64(1):53-9.

9. Leibenluft E. Women with bipolar illness: clinical and research issues. *Am J Psychiatry.* 1996; 153(2):163-73.

10. Lish JD, Dime-Meenan S, Whybrow PC, Price RA, Hirschfeld RM. The National Depressive and Manic-depressive Association (DMDA) survey of bipolar members. *J Affect Disord.* 1994; 31(4):281-94.

11. Delbello MP, Soutullo CA, Strakowski SM. Racial differences in treatment of adolescents with bipolar disorder. *Am J Psychiatry.* 2000; 157(5):837-8.

12. Kirov G, Murray RM. Ethnic differences in the presentation of bipolar affective disorder. *Eur Psychiatry.* 1999; 14(4):199-204.

13. Weissman MM, Gershon ES, Kidd KK, Prusoff BA, Leckman JF, Dibble E, Hamovit J, Thompson WD, Pauls DL, Guroff JJ. Psychiatric disorders in the relatives of probands with affective disorders. The Yale University--National Institute of Mental Health Collaborative Study. *Arch Gen Psychiatry.* 1984; 41(1):13-21.

14. Gershon ES, Hamovit J, Guroff JJ, Dibble E, Leckman JF, Sceery W, Targum SD, Nurnberger JI, Jr., Goldin LR, Bunney WE, Jr.. A family study of schizoaffective, bipolar I, bipolar II, unipolar, and normal control probands. *Arch Gen Psychiatry.* 1982; 39(10):1157-67.

15. Todd RD, Geller B, Neuman R, Fox LW, Hickok J. Increased prevalence of

alcoholism in relatives of depressed and bipolar children. *J Am Acad Child Adolesc Psychiatry.* 1996; 35(6):716-24.

16. Potter W. Biological findings in bipolar disorders, in *Annual Review.* vol 6. Edited by Hales R, American Psychiatric Association, 1987.

17. Bertelsen A, Harvald B, Hauge M. A Danish twin study of manic-depressive disorders. *Br J Psychiatry.* 1977; 130:330-51.

18. Craddock N, Khodel V, Van Eerdewegh P, Reich T. Mathematical limits of multilocus models: the genetic transmission of bipolar disorder. *Am J Hum Genet.* 1995; 57(3):690-702.

19. National Institute of Mental Health: Genetics and Mental Disorders

20. Schwarzkopf SB, Nasrallah HA, Olson SC, Coffman JA, McLaughlin JA. Perinatal complications and genetic loading in schizophrenia: preliminary findings. *Psychiatry Res.* 1989; 27(3):233-9.

21. Hultman CM, Sparen P, Takei N, Murray RM, Cnattingius S. Prenatal and perinatal risk factors for schizophrenia, affective psychosis, and reactive psychosis of early onset: case-control study. *Bmj.* 1999; 318(7181):421-6.

22. Kinney DK, Yurgelun-Todd DA, Tohen M, Tramer S. Pre- and perinatal complications and risk for bipolar disorder: a retrospective study. *J Affect Disord.* 1998; 50(2-3):117-24.

23. Arnold LM. Gender differences in bipolar disorder. *Psychiatr Clin North Am.* 2003; 26(3):595-620.

24. Hunt N, Silverstone T. Does puerperal illness distinguish a subgroup of bipolar patients? *J Affect Disord.* 1995; 34(2):101-7.

25. Bauer M, Whybrow PC. Thyroid hormone, neural tissue and mood modulation. *World J Biol Psychiatry.* 2001; 2(2):59-69.

26. Haggerty JJ, Jr., Evans DL, Golden RN, Pedersen CA, Simon JS, Nemeroff CB. The presence of antithyroid antibodies in patients with affective and nonaffective psychiatric disorders. *Biol Psychiatry.* 1990; 27(1):51-60.

27. Oomen HA, Schipperijn AJ, Drexhage HA. The prevalence of affective disorder and in particular of a rapid cycling of bipolar disorder in patients with abnormal thyroid function tests. *Clin Endocrinol (Oxf).* 1996; 45(2):215-23.

28. Akiskal HS, Djenderedjian AM, Rosenthal RH, Khani MK. Cyclothymic disorder: validating criteria for inclusion in the bipolar affective group. *Am J Psychiatry.* 1977; 134(11):1227-33.

29. Verdoux H, Bourgeois M. Social class in unipolar and bipolar probands and relatives. *J Affect Disord.* 1995; 33(3):181-7.

30. Hunt N, Bruce-Jones W, Silverstone T. Life events and relapse in bipolar affective disorder. *J Affect Disord.* 1992; 25(1):13-20.

31. Johnson SL, Sandrow D, Meyer B, Winters R, Miller I, Solomon D, Keitner G. Increases in manic symptoms after life events involving goal attainment. *J Abnorm Psychol.* 2000; 109(4): 721-7.

32. American Psychiatric Association, American Psychiatric Association Task Force on DSM-IV. *Diagnostic and statistical manual of mental disorders: DSM-IV-TR.* Washington, DC, American Psychiatric Association, 2000.

Chapter 3: Mania & Depression — Elements of Mood in Bipolar Disorder

Mood disorder signifies psychiatric conditions whose predominant features are disturbances in mood, behavior, perception, and cognition.[1] DSM-IV (TR) divides mood disorders into depressive disorders, bipolar disorders, and mood disorders induced by general medical conditions (e.g., drugs or toxins). In addition, the presence of mania/hypomania and one or more depressive episodes differentiate bipolar disorders from depressive disorders.

Chapter 3 at a Glance

Mania in Bipolar Disorder

This section presents the diagnostic criteria, clinical manifestations, associated features, laboratory findings, and clinical course for mania.

Diagnostic Criteria for Mania

Although classified as a syndrome of mood disturbance, mania is also characterized by alterations in behavior, cognition, and perception.[1] Table 3-1. Criteria for Manic Episodes, on the next page, lists the DSM-IV (TR) criteria for a manic episode. Rather than the stereotypical sustained period of euphoria and grandiosity, manic mood symptoms can vary in severity from person to person. Failing to recognize that manic manifestations are not all euphoric can potentially result in a missed diagnosis.

Clinical Manifestations

Symptoms must persist for at least one week to establish a diagnosis of mania. However, if the functional impairment requires hospitalization, DSM-IV (TR) criteria allows for less than one week's duration. Although the expansive, cheerful, or euphoric mood may have an infectious quality for strangers, those who know the patient recognize it as excessive. Table 3-2, on page 3-4, provides examples of each Criterion B symptom.

Mania must significantly impact functional domains, such as:

- Participating in illegal behavior
- Failing to recognize consequences of foolish business decisions
- Exhibiting unusual sexual behavior
- Threatening others

The need for hospitalization or presence of psychotic manifestations also meets Criterion D for marked impairment.

Table 3-1. Criteria for Manic Episodes[2]

A. A distinct period of abnormally and persistently elevated, expansive, or irritable mood, lasting at least one week (or any duration if hospitalization is necessary).

B. During the period of mood disturbance, three (or more) of the following symptoms have persisted (four if the mood is only irritable) and have been present to a significant degree:

   1. Inflated self-esteem or grandiosity
   2. Decreased need for sleep (e.g., feels rested after only three hours of sleep)
   3. More talkative than usual or pressure to keep talking
   4. Flight of ideas or subjective experience that thoughts are racing
   5. Distractibility (i.e., attention too easily drawn to unimportant or irrelevant external stimuli)
   6. Increase in goal-directed activity (either socially, at work or school, or sexually) or psychomotor agitation
   7. Excessive involvement in pleasurable activities that have a high potential for painful consequences (e.g., engaging in unrestrained buying sprees, sexual indiscretions, or foolish business investments)

C. The symptoms do not meet criteria for a Mixed Episode.

D. The mood disturbance is sufficiently severe to cause marked impairment in occupational functioning or in usual social activities or relationships with others, or to necessitate hospitalization to prevent harm to self or others, or there are psychotic features.

E. The symptoms are not due to the direct physiological effects of a substance (e.g., drug of abuse, a medication, or other treatment) or a general medical condition (e.g., hyperthyroidism).

Reprinted with permission of American Psychiatric Association, Diagnostic and Statistical Manual of Mental Disorders, Fourth Edition, Text Revision, Washington, D.C., American Psychiatric Association, 2000.

Table 3-2. Criterion B Manic Features

B Criterion	Example Manifestations
B1 — Inflated Self Esteem	• Attempting to advise public figures or invent a perpetual motion machine • Being irritable/angry with those not convinced of their perceptions of self-worth/grandeur
B2 — Less Need for Sleep	• Waking with excess energy, earlier than usual • Going days without sleep but not exhibiting fatigue
B3 — Pressured Speech	• Speaking in a rapid, loud, difficult-to-understand, ongoing, and difficult-to-interrupt manner • Being prone to monologues outside awareness • Making grandiose gestures or wordplay; singing • Haranguing others, complaining, making hostile statements (when mood is irritable, not expansive)
B4 — Flight of Ideas	• Expressing continuous idea stream in rapid fashion • Switching topics suddenly • Being incoherent or completely disorganized
B5 — Distractibility	• Focusing suddenly on discussion across the room (when in conversation) • Focusing on extraneous stimuli, such as the speaker's hair or clothes, during conversation • Interrupting with irrelevant thoughts
B6— Increase in Goal-Directed Activity	• Writing multiple letters to convey perceptions to friends and public figures • Calling friends or strangers any time, day or night, without concern for intrusion • Starting projects without finishing others
B7— Impulsive Pursuit of High-Risk Activities	• Excessively spending beyond income means • Engaging in unprotected sex with strangers • Driving recklessly

Associated Features

When an individual is manic or experiencing a mixed episode, mood alterations may fluctuate widely — the patient may be euphoric one day and depressed the next. Alternately, a depressed period may last for minutes or hours and may occur simultaneously with mania. As described, mania manifestations include mood alterations as specified in the DSM-IV (TR). Other disturbances in behavior and cognition are often associated with mania as well as indicated in table 3-3 below.

Table 3-3. Manic Features Not Specified in the DSM-IV (TR)[1, 2]

▲ Behavioral symptoms	▲ Cognitive symptoms
◆ Resistance to treatment	◆ Poor insight
◆ Changes in dress, makeup, or appearance to appear more attractive/flamboyant	◆ Confusion
◆ Reckless Gambling	◆ Altered perceptions of smell, hearing, and vision
◆ Antisocial behavior	
◆ Increased libido	
◆ Violence	
◆ Suicide	

Patients may exhibit antisocial behavior, disregard ethical boundaries, physically threaten others, or commit suicide. However, suicidal thoughts are more likely to occur during a mixed than a classic manic episode.[3] See pages 3-12 through 3-14 for a description of mixed episodes.

As mania develops, patients may:

- Abuse substances (e.g., alcohol, stimulants), which may worsen or prolong the episode

- Experience significant impairments in their relationships with spouses or partners, other family members, fellow employees, or supervisors

- Develop cognitive abnormalities (e.g., delusions, hallucinations, and severely disturbed thought processes)

Laboratory Findings

There are no laboratory tests for diagnosing mania. Instead, the diagnosis requires a careful history and psychiatric evaluation. However, a variety of abnormal laboratory findings have been identified in patients with manic episodes, including abnormalities of sleep physiology, dysregulation of the hypothalamic-pituitary-adrenal axis, and dysregulation of neurotransmission and neuroendocrine activity.[2] These physiological changes are not used for diagnostic purposes; they are indicative of the manic state, studied in an effort to further our understanding of the biologic basis of bipolar disorder.

Laboratory findings to pinpoint other causes of manic symptoms are important as symptoms can result from substance abuse (e.g., psychostimulants) and general medical conditions (e.g., hyperthyroidism).

New onset mania in later life is particularly associated with secondary causes and high rates of neurological and medical illnesses. Right hemispheric brain lesions are especially common among neurological causes.

Clinical Course

Although manic episodes can occur in children and seniors, the mean age range for onset is in the late teens to early 20s.[4]

Adolescents are more likely than adults to experience manic episodes with psychotic features.

Approximately 10 to 15 percent of adolescents with a history of recurrent major depressive episodes eventually present with a manic episode.[2]

Onset is usually sudden and may follow psychosocial stressors. Following onset, symptoms rapidly increase over the next several days. Bipolar disorder's clinical course is recurrent: once a manic episode occurs, more than 90 percent of patients will have additional episodes. Without treatment, episodes tend to occur at one- to 2.5-year intervals.

In Carlson's and Goodwin's longitudinal study of mood changes in patients with mania, they describe the following three stages of the most classic presentation:[5]

I.   Mood is predominantly euphoric.

II. Mood becomes irritable, dysphoric, and depressed.

III. Mood is characterized by anxiety, panic, dysphoria, and psychotic symptoms.

An untreated manic episode usually persists from several weeks to months and may end rather abruptly. While the above describes the classical manifestations, in practice there is a wide range of presentations, including first manic symptoms with a dysphoric mood (dysphoric mania/hypomania).[6]

Hypomania in Bipolar Disorder

Hypomania is a mood state manifested by persistently elevated, expansive, or irritable mood. An episode lasts at least four days and is observably different from a patient's non-manic state.

Mood may also be dysphoric. "Mixed or dysphoric hypomanic" describes a patient meeting criteria for hypomania along with sub-threshold depressive symptoms, but one who does not necessarily meet criteria for a depressive episode. Often, mixed hypomania is more common clinically than euphoric hypomania.[7] Using DSM-IV (TR) criteria, the episode would be noted as hypomania, regardless of associated mood symptoms.

Diagnostic Criteria for Hypomania

Alterations in function produced by a hypomanic episode are unequivocal and uncharacteristic of the patient in an asymptomatic state. As defined by the DSM-IV(TR), **hypomanic symptoms are identical to those of mania; however, symptoms are insufficient to produce significant social or**

occupational impairment or require hospitalization (See page 3-3).

Clinical Manifestations

Patients with hypomania experience:

- Distractibility characterized by rapid changes in speech or activities in response to irrelevant external stimuli

- Increased creative/productive, goal-directed activity

- Less need for sleep (manifest by waking earlier)

- Excessive involvement in pleasurable, potentially harmful activities (that are less impulsive/destructive in nature than in mania)

Hypomanic-like episodes, which clearly result from somatic antidepressant treatment (e.g., medication, electroconvulsive therapy, light therapy), should not count toward a bipolar II disorder diagnosis. (See table 3-1.)

Just as with mania, hypomanic manifestations must not be secondary to the effects of drugs, substances of abuse, or a general medical condition. Psychotic symptoms occurring during hypomania automatically define the episode as mania.

Clinical Course

Hypomanic episodes are often briefer than manic ones; they may begin suddenly, reach a plateau within a day or two, and last for a few days, several weeks, or months. Similar to mania, hypomania may end more abruptly than major depressive episodes. Between five and 15 percent of hypomanic patients later develop a manic or mixed episode.[2]

Major Depression in Bipolar Disorder

Dysthymia, depression NOS, and major depression are three types of depressive disorders defined in the DSM-IV (TR)[2] These disorders must be differentiated from the normal processes of grief and bereavement.

Diagnostic Criteria for Major Depression

Dysthymia is a low-intensity, chronic mood disorder of two or more years' duration. Characteristic features include anhedonia, low self esteem, and low energy.

Depression NOS is also referred to as minor depression because the number of symptoms are less than those required for major depression. Interestingly, in primary care practices, 10 to 18 percent of patients with depression NOS will develop a major depressive disorder within a year.[8, 9]

Major depression is the most acutely severe, depressive mood disorder. Table 3-4. below and on the following two pages, lists the diagnostic criteria for major depression, which may be the patient's sole mood disorder (unipolar depression) or a component of a bipolar disorder. While the discussion after table 3-4 of clinical manifestations, associated features, laboratory findings, and clinical course is equally relevant to all major depression forms, it is presented as a foundation for identifying and treating patients with bipolar disorder.

Table 3-4. Criteria for Major Depressive Episodes[2]

A. Five (or more) of the following symptoms have been present during the same 2-week period and represent a change from previous functioning; at least one of the symptoms is either (1) depressed mood or (2) loss of interest or pleasure. **Note:** Do not include symptoms that are clearly due to a general medical condition, or mood-incongruent delusions or hallucinations.

   1. Depressed mood most of the day, nearly every day, as indicated by either subjective report (e.g., feels sad or empty) or observation made by others (e.g., appears tearful). **Note:** in children and adolescents, can be irritable mood.

   2. Markedly diminished interest or pleasure in all, or almost all, activities most of the day, nearly every day

(as indicated by either subjective account or observation made by others).

3. Significant weight loss without a diet, weight gain over five percent of body weight in a month, or decreased/increased appetite nearly *every day*.
Note: in children, consider failure to achieve expected weight gains.

4. Insomnia or hypersomnia nearly every day.

5. Psychomotor agitation or retardation nearly every day (observable by others, not merely subjective feelings of restlessness or being slowed down).

6. Fatigue or loss of energy nearly every day.

7. Feelings of worthlessness or excessive/inappropriate guilt (may be delusional) nearly every day (not merely self-reproach or guilt about being sick).

8. Diminished ability to think, concentrate, or be decisive, nearly every day (either by subjective account or as observed by others).

9. Recurrent thoughts of death (not just fear of dying), recurrent suicidal ideation without a specific plan, or a suicide attempt or a specific plan for committing suicide.

B. The symptoms do not meet criteria for a Mixed Episode (see text).

C. The symptoms cause clinically significant distress or impairment in social, occupational, or other important areas of functioning.

D. The symptoms are not due to the direct physiological effects of a substance (e.g., a drug of abuse, a medication) or a general medical condition (e.g., hypothyroidism).

E. The symptoms are not better accounted for by bereavement (i.e., after the loss of a loved one, the symptoms persist for longer than two months or are characterized by marked functional impairment, morbid preoccupation with worthlessness, suicidal ideation, psychotic symptoms, or psychomotor retardation).

Reprinted with permission of American Psychiatric Association, Diagnostic and Statistical Manual of Mental Disorders, Fourth Edition, Text Revision, Washington, D.C., American Psychiatric Association, 2000.

Clinical Manifestations

Major depression is a change in previous functioning characterized by depressed mood or loss of interest or pleasure for two weeks or more. During this two-week period, patients should present at least five of the nine diagnostic symptoms specified in the DSM-IV (TR).[2]

> *The risk of suicide is particularly high in patients with a previous personal or family suicide history, when depression is accompanied by psychotic features, or with comorbid substance use.*

Laboratory Findings

As many as 90 percent of patients with major depression will have abnormal sleep physiology.[2] Polysomnography may show manifestations described above plus:

- Abnormal rapid eye movement (REM)
- Shifts in non-REM activity away from a first sleep-period
- Increased duration of REM early in sleep

There are a variety of neuroendocrine abnormalities associated with major depression. These include abnormalities of the major neurotransmitter systems as well as disordered hypothalamic-pituitary-adrenal axis (HPAA) physiology (e.g., increased urinary free cortisol levels, failure of dexamethasone to suppress cortisol secretion). In addition, other hormones whose secretory amounts and patterns rely on the hypothalamus and pituitary may have blunted responses to various provocative tests. Functional brain imaging studies during major depressive episodes demonstrate shifts in cortical blood flow and metabolism from the lateral prefrontal cortex to the limbic and paralimbic regions.

Clinical Course

Minor depressive symptoms and anxiety can precede a major depressive episode by weeks or months. Onset of major depression defining symptoms generally occurs over a period of days or weeks. Though age independent, an untreated episode usually lasts four or more months.

Mixed Episodes of Bipolar Disorder

While mania and major depression are often considered to be at opposite ends of the mood spectrum, symptoms of major depression can coexist with those of mania, referred to as a mixed episode.

Diagnostic Criteria for Mixed Episodes

Patients with mixed episodes have symptom duration of at least one week, during which time they meet criteria for both a manic and a major depressive episode. Importantly, the diagnosis is a mixed episode if a patient with mania presents prominent symptoms of a major depressive episode every day for a week or more. (See Table 3-5. Criteria for Mixed Episodes on the next page.)

Presence of mania plus a major depressive episode establishes the diagnosis of a mixed state rather than mania.

A mixed episode diagnosis does not require that the depressive component be present for at least two weeks. Studies indicate that approximately 30 to 40 percent of patients with mania present with mixed symptoms.[10]

Clinical Manifestations

Clinical manifestations of a mixed episode must be of sufficient magnitude that they produce significant functional impairment or lead to hospitalization and are not secondary to drugs or a general medical condition. The presentation often includes agitation, insomnia, appetite dysregulation, suicide ideation, and psychotic features:

Table 3-5. Criteria for Mixed Episodes[2]

A. The criteria are met both for a Manic Episode (see text) and for a Major Depressive Episode (see text) (except for duration) nearly every day during at least a one-week period.

B. The mood disturbance is sufficiently severe to cause marked impairment in occupational functioning or in usual social activities/relationships with others, or to necessitate hospitalization to prevent harm to self or others; or there are psychotic features.

C. The symptoms are not due to the direct physiological effects of a substance (e.g., a drug of abuse, a medication, or other treatment) or a general medical condition (e.g., hyperthyroidism).

Note: Mixed-like episodes that clearly result from somatic antidepressant treatment (e.g., medication, electroconvulsive therapy, light therapy) should not count toward a diagnosis of bipolar I disorder.

Reprinted with permission of American Psychiatric Association, Diagnostic and Statistical Manual of Mental Disorders, Fourth Edition, Text Revision, Washington, D.C., American Psychiatric Association, 2000.

The development of a mixed episode during somatic therapy for depression may be an indication that the patient has a "bipolar diathesis" with an increased risk of later manic, hypomanic, or mixed episodes unrelated to somatic treatments for depression. Debate continues on whether or not development of hypomania during antidepressant treatment indicates a patient will develop bipolar disorders at a later point in time. Studies ongoing should definitely answer this question in the next several years.

Since symptoms of patients with mixed episodes differ significantly from those with pure mania, one must remain alert for the diagnosis. This is particularly important in patients with depression, since hypomania or manic symptoms can co-occur but be episodic and unrecognized by the patient as a change in state.

Laboratory Findings

There are no laboratory findings for diagnosing mixed episodes. Of note are the findings of dysregulation of the hypothalmic-pituitary-adrenal axis, neurotransmitters, and neuroendocrine system that show elements of manic and depressive changes.[2]

Clinical Course

Patients with a mixed episode are more likely to experience depressive delusions and attempt suicide. Failure to recognize the condition can significantly worsen the prognosis.[11–13] Duration of mixed episodes is longer than mania, and relapse may be sooner.

Additionally, differentiation of a mixed episode has therapeutic and prognostic implications. For example:

> If a patient with mixed symptoms is misdiagnosed as having major depression, subsequent antidepressant monotherapy can possibly unmask and exacerbate hypomanic or manic symptoms or induce a manic or hypomanic episode, contributing to treatment refractoriness for future episodes.[14]

This result may also be seen in patients with bipolar disorder, who are treated with antidepressants alone.

The Mood Spectrum

Researchers increasingly define the criteria for bipolar disorder as a spectrum of phenotypic manifestations rather than discrete diagnostic phenotypes. Historically, this transition began with Kraepelin's analysis of manic depressive illness as a distinct clinical entity, included within the "greater part of morbid states termed melancholia."[15] Importantly, however, he differentiated patients with "circular" (manic-depressive) forms of melancholia from those without. Lack of clear boundaries between the various mood disorders led many of Kraepelin's successors to continue to "lump patients with manic depressive illness with those who lacked a manic or hypomanic component.[16]

It was not until the 20th century that Leonhard, and subsequently Angst and Perris, reclassified mood disorders into distinct unipolar and bipolar nosological entities. This "split" of mood disorders persists to date and represents a major advance in the approach to patients with mood disorders.

Subsequently, some investigators broadened bipolarity to a dimensional illness, including a spectrum of non-DSM entities [e.g., borderline bipolar, soft bipolar, and affective temperaments (hyperthymic, cyclothymic, dysthymic, irritable)].[16, 17] Akiskal et. al. emphasized the dimensional nature of the illness by proposing to expand the category to include additional entities and in-between disorders such as bipolar III.[18] The interface of symptoms and "temperament" and implications for course of illness and treatment are an active area of investigation.

The concept of a mood spectrum generally continues to be a topic of debate.

Schizoaffective Disorder: The Continuum Theory

Patients with bipolar disorder can have psychotic symptoms. This leads to a continuum theory that views affective disorders such as major depression, bipolar disorder, and schizophrenia, as a spectrum of disease manifestations, rather than separate disorders with discrete boundaries.[19] Thus, a patient who is predominantly bipolar can have depressive, manic, or psychotic symptoms of variable severity at different time points throughout the course of their disease. Figure 1. Continuum of Affective/Psychotic Disorders on the next page illustrates this concept.

Figure 1. Continuum of Affective/Psychotic Disorders

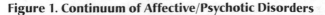

Major Depression	Affective Temperament	Bipolar II	Bipolar I	Schizoaffective	Psychosis

Patients who manifest both affective and psychotic features are classified as schizoaffective. Schizoaffective disorders, as defined by the DSM-IV (TR), consist of a major depressive, manic, or mixed episode accompanied by delusions or hallucinations that meet the criteria for the diagnosis of schizophrenia.[2] However, the psychotic manifestations must last for at least two weeks after full resolution of the mood symptoms, and the disturbance must not be due to substances of abuse, medications, or a general medical disorder.

The symptoms of schizoaffective disorder share significant features with both bipolar disorder and schizophrenia. Therefore, some investigators have proposed that bipolar disorder and schizophrenia are related members of the schizoaffective continuum and that the predominant manifestation is a function of various genetic and environmental factors. A number of findings support the relationship of the two. Both disorders:[20]

- Have a high degree of genetic transmissibility
- Have certain susceptibility markers that can be co-localized to the same chromosome
- Reflect similar abnormalities of neurotransmitter systems
- Respond to treatment with newer generation psychotropic (antipsychotic) medications

It remains to be seen whether greater understanding of the biologic underpinnings will more clearly define a set of discrete disorders or a continuum of disorders.

However, the relationship between the various disorders is still a subject of great debate. Some advocate the unipolar/bipolar dichotomy. Additionally, the genetic basis of these psychiatric diagnoses remains to be fully elucidated.

References

1. Keck PE, Jr., McElroy SL, Arnold LM. Bipolar disorder. *Med Clin North Am.* 2001; 85(3):645-61, ix.

2. American Psychiatric Association, American Psychiatric Association Task Force on DSM-IV. *Diagnostic and statistical manual of mental disorders: DSM-IV-TR.* Washington, DC, American Psychiatric Association, 2000.

3. American Psychiatric Association: Practice guideline for the treatment of patients with bipolar disorder (revision). *Am J Psychiatry.* 2002; 159(4 Suppl):1-50.

4. Faedda GL, Baldessarini RJ, Suppes T, Tondo L, Becker I, Lipschitz DS. Pediatric-onset bipolar disorder: a neglected clinical and public health problem. *Harv Rev Psychiatry.* 1995; 3(4):171-95.

5. Carlson GA, Goodwin FK. The stages of mania. A longitudinal analysis of the manic episode. *Arch Gen Psychiatry.* 1973; 28(2):221-8.

6. Goodwin FK, Jamison KR. *Manic-Depressive Illness.* New York, NY: Oxford University Press, 1990.

7. *Acta Psychiatrica Scandinavica*, Supplementum, No. 423, vol.110, 2004 Poster numbers as follows: Suppes et. al.,: P3.

8 Maier W, Gansicke M, Weiffenbach O. The relationship between major and sub-threshold variants of unipolar depression. J *Affect Disord.* 1997; 45(1-2):41-51.

9. Wells KB, Stewart A, Hays RD, Burnam MA, Rogers W, Daniels M, Berry S, Greenfield S, Ware J. The functioning and well-being of depressed patients. Results from the Medical Outcomes Study. *JAMA.* 1989; 262(7):914-9.

10. McElroy SL, Keck PE, Jr., Pope HG, Jr., Hudson JI, Faedda GL, Swann AC. Clinical and research implications of the diagnosis of dysphoric or mixed mania or hypomania. *Am J Psychiatry.* 1992; 149(12):1633-44.

11. Dilsaver SC, Chen Y W, Swann AC, Shoaib AM, Krajewski KJ. Suicidality in patients with pure and depressive mania. *Am J Psychiatry* 1994; 151(9):1312-5

12. Strakowski SM, McElroy SL, Keck PE, Jr., West SA. Suicidality among patients with mixed and manic bipolar disorder. *Am J Psychiatry.* 1996; 153(5):674-6

13. Strakowski SM, Tohen M, Stoll A. Comorbidity in mania at first hospitalization. *Am J Psychiatry.* 1992; 149:554-556.

14. Kupfer DJ, Carpenter LL, Frank E. Possible role of antidepressants in precipitating mania and hypomania in recurrent depression. *Am J Psychiatry.* 1988; 145(7):804-8.

15. Kraepelin E. Manic-depressive insanity and paranoia, in *Manic-depressive insanity and paranoia.* Edited by Barclay R, Robertson G. Edinburgh: E & S Livingston, 1921.

16 Cassano GB, Frank E, Miniati M, Rucci P, Fagiolini A, Pini S, Shear MK, Maser JD. Conceptual underpinnings and empirical support for the mood spectrum. *Psychiatr Clin North Am.* 2002; 25(4):699-712.

17. Angst J. The emerging epidemiology of hypomania and bipolar II disorder. *J Affect Disord.* 1998; 50(2-3):143-51.

18. Akiskal HS, Pinto O. The evolving bipolar spectrum. Prototypes I, II, III, and IV. *Psychiatr Clin North Am.* 1999; 22(3):517-34, vii.

19. Lapierre YD. Schizophrenia and manic-depression: separate illnesses or a continuum? *Can J Psychiatry.* 1994; 39(9 Suppl 2):S59-64.

20. Moller HJ. Bipolar disorder and schizophrenia: distinct illnesses or a continuum? *J Clin Psychiatry.* 2003; 64 Suppl 6:23-7; discussion 28.

Chapter 4: Diagnosis of Bipolar Disorder and Its Subtypes

Two main types of mood disorders — major depressive (unipolar) and manic depressive (bipolar) — each have distinctive genetic and clinical characteristics. This chapter describes a diagnostic approach for patients with bipolar disorder.

While the previous chapter focused on the characteristics and clinical manifestations of each element of bipolar disorder— mania, hypomania, depression, and mixed episodes — this chapter will focus on helping the clinician determine which form of what symptom subgroup exists among patients presenting in the clinical setting.

Chapter 4 at a Glance

The DSM-IV (TR) lists four bipolar disorders in its bipolar category:[1]

- Bipolar I (divided into six criteria sets to specify the type of the most recent episode)
- Bipolar II
- Cyclothymia
- Bipolar disorder not otherwise specified (NOS)

Bipolar II, cyclothymia, and bipolar NOS are without separate episode-type criteria sets.

However, a number of other criteria sets exist that can apply

Chapter 3 addresses diagnostic criteria for mania, (pages 3-2 to 3-3), and depression (pages 3-9 to 3-11). Hypomanic criteria are identical to those of mania, but don't cause social/ occupational impairment or hospitalization.

to all bipolar disorders and help to provide a comprehensive picture of the illness. For example, one of the bipolar disorder courses *specified by* DSM-IV (TR) is rapid cycling: a distinctive pattern that, despite its specific therapeutic and prognostic features, is *not* currently categorized as a specific subtype of bipolar disorder.

Bipolar I Disorder

The diagnosis of bipolar I disorder requires the presence of at least one manic episode, with or without a history of a prior major depressive episode.[1] (See table 1 below.)

Table 4-1. Diagnostic Criteria for Bipolar I Disorder, Single Manic Episode

A. Presence of only one manic episode and no past major depressive episodes. If this is the first manic presentation and there is a history of major depressive episode(s) in past, then the diagnosis is bipolar disorder, most recent episode manic.

B. The manic episode is not better accounted for by schizoaffective disorder and is not superimposed on Schizophrenia, Schizophreniform disorder, Delusional disorder, or Psychotic disorder Not Otherwise Specified.

Reprinted with permission of American Psychiatric Association, Diagnostic and Statistical Manual of Mental Disorders, Fourth Edition, Text Revision, Washington, D.C., American Psychiatric Association, 2000.

Bipolar II Disorder

Bipolar II disorder diagnosis requires the presence of at least one hypomanic episode, with a history of at least one prior major depressive episode.[1] (See table 2 below and chapter 3.) There should be no history of a manic or mixed episode, since the presence of either is diagnostic for bipolar I, not bipolar II, disorder.

Table 4-2. Diagnostic Criteria for Bipolar II Disorder

A. Presence (or history) of one or more major depressive episodes.

B. Presence (or history) of at least one hypomanic episode.

C. There has never been a manic episode or a mixed episode.

D. The mood symptoms in Criteria A and B are not better accounted for by schizoaffective disorder and are not superimposed on Schizophrenia, Schizophreniform disorder, Delusional disorder, or Psychotic disorder Not Otherwise Specified.

E. The symptoms cause clinically significant distress or impairment in social, occupational, or other important areas of functioning.

Reprinted with permission of American Psychiatric Association, Diagnostic and Statistical Manual of Mental Disorders, Fourth Edition, Text Revision, Washington, D.C., American Psychiatric Association, 2000.

As described in chapter 3, hypomania differs from mania in severity: as a less severe manifestation. By definition, it does not produce marked functional impairment or require hospitalization. While hypomania can be a transitional stage between euthymia and mania in patients with bipolar I disorder, hypomania is considered a stable ceiling of manic symptoms in bipolar II disorder. That is, for patients with bipolar II disorder, hypomanic symptoms during the episode do not mean the patient will develop mania. Whereas for bipolar I, hypomania is an unstable state that may herald the development of mania.

Table 4-3, on the next page, shows the associated features and clinical course of bipolar II disorder similar to those of bipolar I disorder.

Because bipolar disorder is under-identified, symptoms of mania or hypomania should be sought in any patient with apparent unipolar major depressive episode. Since manic and hypomanic symptoms may be pleasurable, patients may only seek medical advice at the time of a major depressive episode. Patients may be unable to remember manic or hypomanic episodes as such or may fail to differentiate them from normal mood states.

DSM-IV(TR) doesn't distinguish between euphoric and mixed or dysphoric hypomania (coded as hypomania, regardless of associated mood symptoms). However, many patients, when hypomanic, present with concurrent depressive symptoms ("dysphoric hypomania"), making differentiation from ongoing depressive symptoms difficult and often unidentified as hypomania. While many bipolar II patients may have a history of hypomanic episodes, what they may experience the majority of the time is more transient hypomanic or dysphoric hypomanic symptoms.

Table 4-3. Clinical Features of Bipolar I and II Disorders

Clinical Feature	Bipolar I	Bipolar II
Gender	F = M*	F>M*
Mania	Yes	No
Hypomania	Yes (as a transitional state)	Yes
Major depressive disorder Required for Initial Diagnosis	No	Yes
Psychotic symptoms[1]	Yes, can occur during either phase	Does not occur during hypomanic phase[1] Less common in major depressive episode than with bipolar I
Completed Suicide[2]	Same	Same
Rapid Cycling Incidence[3]	Same	Same
Relationship of manic/hypomanic episodes to major depressive episode[4]	Same	Same
Interval Between episodes	May decrease with age**	May decrease with age**

Notes: [1]Psychotic symptoms during hypomania move episode to be defined as mania. [2]Completed Suicide = 10% to 15%. [3]Rapid Cycling = 10% to 20%. [4]Relationship of manic/hypomanic episodes to major depressive episodes — 60% to 70% immediately before or after.

* In males, the first episode is more likely to be manic; in females, the first episode is more likely to be depression. Males experience more mania episodes throughout the lifetime of the disorder while females experience more depressive episodes

** *Between episodes, patients experience significantly reduced symptoms; however, many have residual, sub-syndromal symptoms that, if not treated, can lead to functional impairment.*

Cyclothymia

Cyclothymia is a chronic, fluctuating mood disorder with numerous hypomanic and mild depressive symptoms.[1] (See table 4-4 on the next page.) Both the hypomanic and depressive symptoms are of insufficient number, severity, pervasiveness, or duration to meet full criteria for a major depressive or hypomanic episode.

Cyclothymic disorder is usually chronic and as many as 50 percent of patients will subsequently develop bipolar I or bipolar II disorder.[1] Importantly, the development of major depressive, hypomanic or manic symptoms after two years of cyclothymic manifestations does not negate the diagnosis of cyclothymic disorder; instead, patients are diagnosed with cyclothymic disorder plus the other major mood disorder.

Bipolar NOS

The bipolar NOS category is a residual diagnostic category for disorders with bipolar features that do not meet criteria for bipolar I, bipolar II, or cyclothymic disorder. A patient might experience multiple hypomanic episodes without inter-current major depressive episodes, or hypomanic and depressive symptoms may be too infrequent to qualify the patient for a cyclothymic diagnosis. In some instances, the NOS qualifier will be used while the clinician attempts to determine if the disorder is truly primary or is secondary to substances of abuse or a medical condition.

Diagnostic Specifiers for Bipolar Disorder

Diagnostic specifiers increase diagnostic specificity, aid in treatment selection, and improve prognostic accuracy. In addition, they also can improve the homogeneity of subgroups in clinical trials of bipolar disorder treatments and, thus, data analysis.

Table 4-4. Diagnostic Criteria for Cyclothymic Disorder

A. For at least 2 years, the presence of numerous periods with hypomanic symptoms and numerous periods with depressive symptoms that do not meet criteria for a hypomanic or a major depressive episode. **Note:** In children and adolescents, the duration must be at least 1 year.

B. During the above 2-year period (1 year in children and adolescents), the patient has not been without the symptoms in Criterion A for more than 2 months at a time.

C. No major depressive episode, manic episode, or mixed episode has been present during the first 2 years of the disturbance. **Note:** After the initial 2 years (1 year in children and adolescents) of cyclothymic disorder, there may be superimposed manic or mixed episodes (in which case both bipolar I disorder and cyclothymic disorder may be diagnosed) or hypomanic and major depressive episodes (in which case both bipolar II disorder and cyclothymic disorder may be diagnosed).

D. The symptoms in Criterion A are not better accounted for by schizoaffective disorder and are not superimposed on Schizophrenia, Schizophreniform disorder, Delusional disorder, or Psychotic disorder Not Otherwise Specified.

E. The symptoms are not due to the direct physiological effects of a substance, e.g., a drug of abuse, a medication, or a general medical condition e.g., hyperthyroidism.

F. The symptoms cause clinically significant distress or impairment in social, occupational, or other important areas of functioning.

Reprinted with permission of American Psychiatric Association, Diagnostic and Statistical Manual of Mental Disorders, Fourth Edition, Text Revision, Washington, D.C., American Psychiatric Association, 2000.

Specifiers Related to Episode, Onset, and Course

Bipolar disorder specifiers for the episode, onset, and course of the disorder have been developed and are listed in the DSM-IV (TR).[1] (See tables 4-5a, b, and c, below and on page 4-9, for each category's appropriate diagnostic specifiers.)

Table 4–5a. Bipolar Disorder Specifiers for Episode

Specifier	Comments
Severity	• Mild, moderate, or severe
Psychotic	• With or without psychotic symptoms
Remission	• In partial or full remission
Chronic	• Applied to mood disorder with a major depressive episode (i.e., major depression; bipolar I, most recent episode depressed; or, bipolar II, depressed)
Catatonic	• Motoric immobility or excessive purposeless motor activity • Extreme negativism • Peculiarities of voluntary movement • Echolalia or echopraxia
Melancholic	• Near complete absence of the capacity for pleasure • Present at nadir • Distinctively different than sadness or non-melancholic depression
Atypical Depression	• Mood reactivity—mood brightens in response to positive events • Significant weight gain or increase in appetite • Hypersomnia • Heavy, leaden feelings in arms and/or legs • Long-standing; impairment resulting from sensitivity to rejection

Table 4-5b. Bipolar Disorder Specifiers for Onset

Specifier	Comments
Post-partum	• Onset of major mood disorder within 4 weeks post-partum

Table 4-5c. Bipolar Disorder Specifiers for Course

Specifier	Comments
With or Without Inter-episode Recovery	• With full-recovery • Without full-recovery
Seasonal Pattern*	• With or without • Regular, temporal relationship between major mood disorder onset and season • Seasonal, full-remission • Two seasonal major depressive episodes in 2 years • Seasonal major depressive episodes significantly outnumber nonseasonal ones during one's lifetime
Rapid Cycling	• Applied to bipolar I or II disorder • ≥4 episodes of mood disturbance in previous 12 months that meet criteria for major mood episode • Episodes have partial or full remission for at least 2 months, or there is a switch to an episode of opposite polarity

* DSM-IV (TR) discusses a seasonal depressive pattern only, but it is well recognized that seasonal patterns exist for hypomania and mania for some patients.

Reprinted with permission of American Psychiatric Association, Diagnostic and Statistical Manual of Mental Disorders, Fourth Edition, Text Revision, Washington, D.C., American Psychiatric Association, 2000.

Special Notes on Rapid Cycling

Rapid cycling is an important course specifier for patients (with an established diagnosis of bipolar I or II disorder), who experience four or more mood episodes within a 12-month period that are either:

- Discrete, (i.e., demarcated by a partial or full remission of at least two months' duration); or

- Characterized by a switch to an episode of opposite polarity.

Any subtype with a manic or hypomanic component is not considered to have "cycled." Thus, the disorders remain in the same pole when a mixed episode immediately follows a manic one, despite depressive symptomatology in the mixed episode. Another example would be severe depression changing to mild depression; symptoms would still be occurring at the same pole, and thus would not be considered to have switched.

Although bipolar disorder is gender neutral, women are two to nine times more likely to have a rapid cycling course than men. Despite the gender bias, rapid cycling episodes appear to be unrelated to the reproductive cycle or stage.

A rapid cycling course can be intermittent or persistent and can occur at any time during illness course. It is more common in patients with a variety of medical disorders, including hypothyroidism, neurological conditions, and mental retardation.[1]

Diagnosing the Patient with Bipolar Disorder

The history and mental status examination are the most important tools for diagnosing a patient with bipolar disorder.

Although these elements have been formalized, the diagnostic process really begins when the patient first walks into the office. The office staff may give the first indication that the patient has a mood disorder when they report that the patient is "talking a mile a minute," "cannot sit still," or is "sitting slumped in their seat, teary-eyed." Attention should be paid to the patient's general appearance: are they well groomed and dressed appropriately? Do they talk to themselves or appear to be hallucinating?

Questioning the Patient in the Initial Interview

In the course of the initial interview, it can be helpful to first ask questions in an open-ended fashion so that the physician has the opportunity to determine the basis for the visit.

> *Patients with a rapid cycling course comprise approximately 10 to 20 percent of the overall population of patients with bipolar disorder.*[1]

As the interview progresses, questions may become more focused to obtain specific information, such as dates of symptom onset and duration of episodes. Since patients with psychiatric illnesses may not always be the best historians, a definite diagnosis of bipolar disorder cannot always be made from patient self-report. In fact, lack of insight is often a component of bipolar disorder. Therefore, it is often important to elicit supplemental and corroborating information from the patient's family members, significant others, and associates.

Evaluating Symptom Presentation

Those with bipolar disorder often present as depressed. Less often, they present with mixed or dysphoric hypomania (co-occurring depressive manifestations with hypomania), or mania. The following describes important diagnostic considerations for each presentation.

The Patient with Mania

The seven "B" criteria (as discussed in chapter 3) for the diagnosis of mania/hypomania can be recalled by the mnemonic DIGFAST. (See Table 4-6. DIGFAST on the next page.) A manic/hypomanic disorder is present if three (if euphoric) or four (if irritable) DIGFAST criteria are present.

With mania, unlike hypomania, significant dysfunction exists in the social and/or occupational domain. Thus, a patient with the appropriate number of DIGFAST criteria who is not impaired or psychotic, or who does not require hospitalization, has a hypomanic episode. Furthermore, manic symptoms must be present for at least one week (unless hospitalization is necessary), while hypomania can be diagnosed after only four days of DIGFAST symptoms. Hypomania with psychotic features automatically is defined as a manic episode.

Table 4-6. DIGFAST Mnemonic For Mania/Hypomania[1]

- **DISTRACTIBILITY**: Inability to maintain one's focus on tasks for an extended duration

- **INSOMNIA**: Decreased need for sleep coupled with increased energy in manic/hypomanic patients (must be differentiated from the insomnia of major depressive episode)

- **GRANDIOSITY**: Unrealistic, high self-confidence or delusional

- **FLIGHT** of Ideas: Racing thoughts

- **ACTIVITIES**: Increased goal-directed activities that may be appropriate in their nature, but clearly excessive, occurring in social, sexual, school, or workplace domains

- **SPEECH**: Significantly more talkative compared to periods of euthymia

- **THOUGHTLESSNESS**: Dysfunctional, self-centered activities, such as: spending sprees, unprotected sex with strangers, and other impulsive behaviors

The Patient with Mixed or Dysphoric Hypomania

Mixed or dysphoric hypomania is a term used to describe co-occurring depressive symptoms that do not meet criteria for a depressive episode in a patient with symptoms of hypomania or mania. Since this diagnosis has significant prognostic and

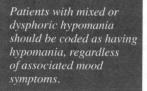

Patients with mixed or dysphoric hypomania should be coded as having hypomania, regardless of associated mood symptoms.

therapeutic implications, the clinician must consider the possibility in a patient presenting with either depressive or manic symptoms — patients with mixed (dysphoric) features may be less likely to recover, more likely to relapse sooner, and are at an increased risk of suicide.[2] In fact, if the patient presenting with bipolar disorder has significant suicidal ideation, the odds are increased that they are dysphoric.[3] Patients with dysphoric hypomania may be less likely to respond to lithium and, especially, to antidepressant therapy.[4, 5] Instead, they are more likely to need other types of medication treatment (e.g., anticonvulsants and atypical antipsychotics).

The Patient with Depression

A bipolar disorder diagnosis should be considered for any patient presenting with a major depressive episode. Criteria for a major depressive episode can be recalled with the mnemonic SAD-A-FACES as shown on the following page.

A single manic or hypomanic episode changes a diagnosis from one of major depressive episodes to bipolar disorder, most recent episode depressed.

Table 4-7. SAD-A-FACES
Mnemonic for Depression[6]

SAD

- **S**LEEP Disturbance (insomnia/hypersomnia)
- **A**PPETITE or weight change
- **D**YSPHORIA "bad mood"

-A-

- **A**NHEDONIA

FACES

- **F**ATIGUE
- **A**GITATION/motor retardation
- **C**ONCENTRATION diminished
- **E**STEEM (low)/guilt
- **S**UICIDE/thoughts of death

A primary major depressive episode is either bipolar or unipolar. Patients with a unipolar major depressive episode do not have a history of mania or hypomania — the patient is either depressed or euthymic and does not experience wide mood swings. The possibility of a dysphoric hypomanic period or "energized depression" must be explored. Therefore, before a diagnosis of unipolar depression can be made, both secondary depression and bipolar disorder must be ruled out. Additionally, many patients with bipolar depression will have an "atypical" presentation, particularly seen as increased sleeping and appetite.

Assessing Medical History

A patient's history should rule out the possibility that the symptoms result from use of a substance or medication, or from a general medical disorder. Chapter 5 covers details on physiological causes for symptoms presented by the patient that must be differentiated from bipolar disorder. Some physiological causes to rule out are:

> *Research has also shown that the abuse of some drugs, including cocaine and corticosteroids, can cause bipolar-like syndromes.*

- **Embolic Stroke**, which occurs typically in an elderly individual. For example, parietal lobe strokes have been implicated in both the development of depression and mania for some individuals.

- **Thyroid conditions**, which include hyperthyroidism (an excess of thyroid hormone), which can cause manic-like symptoms or hypothyroidism (decreased thyroid hormone), which cause depression-like symptoms. Blood tests will indicate changes in hormone levels. Both conditions are associated with physical symptoms not usually observed in patients with bipolar disorder (e.g., elevated heart rate and blood pressure in hyperthyroidism and sensitivity to temperature change and skin bruises and tears in hypothyroidism).

- **Temporal lobe epilepsy**, which is associated with many of the same symptoms that can be seen in bipolar disorder — no coincidence since one of the main brain structures implicated in bipolar disorder is the brain's temporal lobe.

- **Neoplastic or cancer syndromes**, which can also be associated with some patients' change in usual presentation and development of bipolar-like symptoms.

Table 4-8. General Medical/Neurological Disorders that Can Present with Mood Symptoms

▲ **Metabolic Conditions**
- ◆ Vitamin B12 deficiency
- ◆ Porphyria
- ◆ Post-operative state
- ◆ Electrolyte abnormalities

▲ **Endocrinopathies**
- ◆ Hyperthyroidism/hypothyroidism
- ◆ Hyperparathyroidism/hypoparathyroidism
- ◆ Adrenocortical dysfunction (Addison's Disease, Cushing's Disease)

▲ **Infections**
- ◆ Encephalitis
- ◆ Human immunodeficiency virus
- ◆ Hepatitis (A, B)
- ◆ Epstein Barr (Infectious Mononucleosis)
- ◆ Neurosyphilis
- ◆ Influenza
- ◆ Lyme disease

▲ **Coronary Heart Disease**

▲ **Autoimmune/Connective Tissue Disorders**
- ◆ Systemic lupus erythematosus
- ◆ Fibromyalgia

▲ **Malignancy**
- ◆ Carcinoma of the pancreas
- ◆ Multiple myeloma (calcium-related)

▲ **Neurodegenerative Diseases**
- ◆ Parkinson's disease
- ◆ Huntington's disease
- ◆ Alzheimer's disease

▲ **Demyelinating Diseases**
- ◆ Multiple sclerosis

▲ **Other CNS Disease**
- ◆ Stroke
- ◆ Right hemispheric lesions

- ◆ Closed-head injury
- ◆ Normal pressure hydrocephalus
- ◆ Cerebral sarcoidosis
- ◆ Tuberous sclerosis
- ◆ Familial cerebellar disease
- ◆ Idiopathic basal ganglia calcification
- ◆ Subcortical gray matter heterotopia

▲ **Drugs**
- ◆ Adrenal cortical steroids
- ◆ Isoniazid
- ◆ Disulfiram

The laboratory work-up of a young to middle-aged patient, in the absence of medical or neurological findings by history and examination, are in part directed by the need to rule out a primary cause of the manic syndrome and by the anticipated medical treatment. Important measures to obtain include:

- Baseline complete blood count (CBC)
- Thyroid hormone assay (TSH, T3, and T4)
- Fasting glucose and lipid profile (total cholesterol and HDL-C)
- Hepatic function tests (transaminase levels)
- Renal function test (creatinine and BUN)

Past history of head injury should always be part of a medical assessment for the possibility of bipolar disorder because head injury in and of itself can be either a causal or an aggravating factor for bipolar symptoms. Given that many untreated patients with bipolar disorder have low impulse control and a tendency to engage in risky behavior, the possibility for head injury becomes particularly pertinent. Physicians should consider a brain scan for those patients who have never had one.

Assessing Psychiatric History

A major goal in examining the psychiatric history of a patient with possible bipolar disorder is to determine if the patient has had at least one manic or hypomanic episode some time in their life.

The history of the present illness should include a chronology of events related to the chief complaint, including recent exacerbations, remissions, and responses to therapeutic interventions. It is helpful to ask if changes in mood have affected their life at home, work, or school. For example, has periodic irritability impacted work and/or home environment and relationships?

The presence of any past psychiatric episodes or care may provide a clue to the diagnosis. Since patients with bipolar disorder may have previously been treated with antidepressants, the following clues will help the physician identify bipolar disorder in patients treated with antidepressants:

- "Refractory depression," an initial rapid response followed by increasing drug-resistance

- Illness course worsened by antidepressant therapy

- Rapid mood swings (cycling) in response to the medication

- The need for combination therapy with an antidepressant plus a mood stabilizer such as lithium

Patients with bipolar disorder are more likely than the general population to have problems with the legal system. Inquiries should be made about arrests (including driving under the influence), jail time, probation, upcoming court dates, etc. Additionally, the use of alcohol and substances should be carefully explored given the high lifetime prevalence of alcohol and substance use disorders in patients with bipolar disorder.

Psychoactive substances can induce secondary mood disorders. The presence of substance use disorder does not rule out a diagnosis of mood disorder. However, if episodes of abnormal mood exclusively develop during episodes of substance abuse, the diagnosis changes to substance-induced mood disorder. Substance-induced mood disorder must be differentiated from the use of substances to ameliorate affective symptoms (see chapter 5, pages 5-2 through 5-7, for information on substance abuse, differential diagnosis, and comorbidity). A careful medication history must also be taken (e.g., both corticosteroids and L-Dopa can induce secondary mania).

Assessing Family History

Because bipolar disorder has a strong genetic basis, it is important to question the patient about a family history of mood disorders. This should include focused questions about the presence of specific hypomanic, manic, or depressive symptoms in family members—particularly first-degree relatives. Other clues may be suicide attempts or hospitalizations for mental illness. Where a history of suicide exists for family members, the patient can have a higher suicide risk.

The family history should also inquire about the presence of psychiatric comorbidities associated with bipolar disorder and the use of mental health medications by family members. For example, a relative may have been identified as alcoholic and having problems with anger versus being identified as having bipolar disorder and substance abuse. A social history must also be included as it may reveal changes in interpersonal relationships that result from bipolar symptoms or interpersonal difficulties secondary to a comor-bidity commonly associated with bipolar disorder.

Chapter 5 describes comorbid disorders in detail.

Suicide and Homicide Risk

Patients with bipolar disorder have 10 to 15 percent lifetime suicide rates.[7] Every patient who may have bipolar disorder or describes depressive symptoms should be asked about suicidal ideation, plans or preparations for suicide, and intent to act on those plans. They should also be asked about access to medications or firearms that may be used to commit suicide. In most instances, suicide attempts are associated with depressive manifestations, either during a major depressive or mixed episode.

While homicidal behavior is uncommon, clinicians should also query a patient as to aggressive impulses towards others. A past history of aggressive behavior or legal difficulties as well as aggressive behavior associated with alcohol or other substance use should be explored.

References

1. American Psychiatric Association, American Psychiatric Association Task Force on DSM-IV. *Diagnostic and statistical manual of mental disorders: DSM-IV-TR*. Washington, DC, American Psychiatric Association, 2000.

2. Montano CB. Recognition and treatment of depression in a primary care setting. *J Clin Psychiatry*. 1994;55(Suppl):18-34.

3. Keller MB, Lavori PW, Coryell W, Endicott J, Mueller TI. Bipolar I: a five-year prospective follow-up. *J Nerv Ment Dis*. 1993; 181(4):238-45.

4. Goldberg JF, Garno JL, Leon AC, Kocsis JH, Portera L. Association of recurrent suicidal ideation with nonremission from acute mixed mania. *Am J Psychiatry*. 1998; 155(12):1753-5.

5. Arnold LM, McElroy SL, Keck PE, Jr.. The role of gender in mixed mania. *Compr Psychiatry*. 2000; 41(2):83-7.

6. Bauer MS, Whybrow PC, Gyulai L, Gonnel J, Yeh HS. Testing definitions of dysphoric mania and hypomania: prevalence, clinical characteristics and inter episode stability. *J Affect Disord*. 1994; 32(3):201-11.

7. American Psychiatric Association: Practice guideline for the treatment of patients with bipolar disorder (revision). *Am J Psychiatry*. 2002; 159(4 Suppl):1-50.

Chapter 5: Differential Diagnosis & Comorbidity

Because of the range of mood presentations of episodes in bipolar illness and the highly individual course of the disorder from one patient to another, accurate diagnosis can be challenging. Comorbid disorders as well as those medical and psychiatric conditions with similar symptoms further complicate diagnosis.

This chapter takes a three-fold approach to these diagnostic dilemmas by addressing:

1. How can bipolar disorder and conditions that present similar symptoms be differentiated?
2. What disorders tend to be comorbid with bipolar disorder?
3. What treatment approaches exist for treating bipolar disorder and comorbid conditions?

Chapter 5 at a Glance

Conditions Relevant to Differential Diagnosis

A variety of general medical and psychiatric conditions can present similar symptoms to bipolar disorder.

General Medical and Neurological Conditions

General medical and neurological conditions can produce alterations in mood that must be differentiated from manifestations of bipolar disorder. In this type of secondary mood disorder, the mood disturbance is determined to be the direct neurobiological consequence of a specific, often chronic, general medical/neurological disorder. See table 4.8 on pages 4-16 through 4-17 for medical conditions that can present as mood symptoms.

Psychiatric Disorders

Psychiatric disorders that produce mood disturbances to be differentiated from those of bipolar disorder include:

- Substance-related disorders
- Major depressive episode
- Dysthymic disorder
- Schizophrenia and schizoaffective disorder
- Attention Deficit Hyperactivity Disorder (ADHD)
- Impulse-control disorders
- Psychotic disorder NOS

Substance-Related Disorders

Of all disorders with symptoms similar to bipolar disorder, probably substance-related disorders are the most common. The basis for this association may be one or more of the following:

1. Patients at risk for substance abuse disorder may also be at risk for bipolar disorder.

2. Substance abuse disorder may be genetically linked to the risk for bipolar disorder.

3. Chronic substance abuse may induce the development of mood symptoms and episodes.

4. Bipolar disorder is associated with poor impulse control, which can lead to more substance use.

5. Patients may be self-medicating affective symptoms.

Substance is a term used to refer to drugs of abuse, medications, and toxins. Those substances that, especially when abused, can cause bipolar-like (manic and/or depressive) symptoms include alcohol, cocaine and other stimulants, sedatives/hypnotics, and opioids. Substance-related disorders include substance dependence and withdrawal disorders, substance abuse, and substance intoxication. (See Table 5.1. Substance-Induced Mood Disorders, Intoxication/Withdrawal below.)

Table 5 1. Substance Induced Mood Disorders (Intoxication/Withdrawal)

Substance	Mood Swings	Irritability	Mania	Depression
Ethanol (Alcohol)	■	■		■
Stimulants	■	■	■	■
Sedatives/ Hypnotics		■		■
Opioids				■
Inhalants				■
Corticosteroids	■	■	■	■

Table 5-2 below summarizes typical clues for differentiating substance-related mood disorders from primary mood disorders.

Table 5-2. Differential Clues to Substance-Related Mood Disorders

▲ **Suspect Substance-Related Mood Disorder if:**
- ◆ History of substance abuse
- ◆ Manifestations are typical of physiological/behavioral alterations associated with the substance
- ◆ Onset and offset of clinical features temporally-related to substance use
- ◆ Features and course are atypical for mood disorder

▲ **Suspect Primary Mood Disorder if:**
- ◆ Symptoms persist more than two to four weeks after substance discontinuation
- ◆ Dose of substance unlikely to produce clinical manifestations
- ◆ History of mood disorders in first-degree relatives
- ◆ History of prior mood episodes unrelated to substance use

Alcohol Use

Alcohol, a CNS depressant, can potentiate the inhibitory actions of GABA as well as the receptor function of the excitatory amino acid NMDA. Because it also acts on a variety of other neurotransmitter systems, mood symptoms are common. Depression and insomnia that may suggest a major depressive disorder frequently accompany alcohol dependence and may even precede it.[1] Those with mild alcohol intoxication may have a sense of well being and a bright expansive mood as ethanol levels rise. Following this period, depressive and/or anxiety symptoms may worsen.

Stimulant Use

Stimulants producing altered mood states that mimic bipolar disorder manifestations include:

- • Cocaine

- Amphetamines

- Methamphetamine

- Methylenedioxymetham-
  phetamine (MDMA)

> *In patients with bipolar disorder who have a co-occurring substance abuse disorder, the diagnoses would be bipolar disorder and the specific substance abuse disorder.*

Table 5-3, on the following page, presents the typical symptoms of substance abuse for these drugs as well as drug "street" names.

Intoxication with Sedatives and Hypnotics

Sedatives, such as the benzodiazepines that have a rapid onset (e.g., diazepam and alprazolam) tend to be BOTH popular among drug abusers seeking the drugs' ability to produce a "high" AND the most commonly prescribed drugs in the world.[2] Barbiturates and non-benzodiazepine medications can also produce similar symptoms. Withdrawal symptoms mimic mania (e.g., anxiety, agitation, and delirium). Methaqualone ("Quaalude," "Lude"), classified as a schedule I substance since the early 1980s, is easily synthesized and sold for its psychoactive effects. Symptoms of intoxication and withdrawal are similar to those of other sedative/hypnotics. Table 5-4 on page 5-7 covers sedative abuse.

Opioid Abuse

As drugs of abuse, opioid intoxication can produce euphoria, tranquility, and other mood changes believed to be the effects of the drugs on mesolimbic dopaminergic pathways and the nucleus accumbens.[3] Intoxication can also produce CNS and respiratory depression. Withdrawal may be accompanied by dysphoria and irritability.

Although heroin is the most common opiate abused, significantly more potent designer derivatives of fentanyl and meperidine are manufactured in illegal laboratories.[4] Designer opioid intoxication typically shows up in a patient with a negative urinary opioid screen and mood alterations.

Table 5-3. Stimulants and Possible Symptoms

	Possible Symptoms	Impact
Cocaine and Amphetamines (crack, coke, speed, ice, meth)	• Intensive feelings of well being • Euphoria • Racing thoughts • Pressured speech • Hyperactivity • Increased sexual activity • Impulsive behavior • Grandiosity • Paranoia • Insomnia	• Inhibits dopamine reuptake into the nerve terminals via the dopamine transporter in the mesolimbic dopaminergic system and stimulates dopamine and other catecholamine release from pre-synaptic terminals[5] • May induce periods of depression/decreased energy after manic/hypomanic symptoms
MDMA (ecstasy, XTC, M&M)*	• Euphoria • Empathy • Enhanced sociability • Increased energy • Memory loss (73%) • Depression (65%) • Impaired concentration (70%) • Poor sleep (52%) • Anxiety (60%) • Weight loss (48%) • Tremors (30%) • Paranoid psychosis (for typical recreational use over a long time) that is clinically indistinguishable from schizophrenia (reversible after patient is drug-free for an extended period)[4]	• May induce periods of depression/decreased energy after manic/hypomanic symptoms • Clinical implications are based on studies that suggest toxicity to serotonergic neurons, cells implicated in the pathophysiology of depression.[2] • Party-goers are known to take MDMA several times during an evening/night, which has been associated with structural abnormalities of the CNS[6]

Table 5-4. Sedatives and Possible Symptoms

	Possible Symptoms	Impact
Gamma hydroxybutyrate (Easy Lay, Georgia Home Boy, and Liquid Ecstasy, "date rape" drug)	• Mood alterations (e.g., euphoria) • Hallucinations • Amnesia • Intensified effects of other drugs	• A CNS depressant • "Date rape" drug
Flunitrazepam (Rohypnol) (La Roche, Roofies, Mexican Valium, and "date rape" drug)	• Euphoria • Depersonalization, • Emotional withdrawal inebriation • Decreased pain perception • Manic-like and psychotic symptoms (dose-dependent)	• No longer available in U.S., but smuggled in from other countries • Unlike other benzodiazepines, it is not detected by standard enzyme multiplied immunoassay technique (EMIT) procedure as Ketamine and PCP analogs may also escape detection in assays designed to identify PCP

Corticosteroid Use

Corticosteroids are widely used to treat a variety of inflammatory and immune-mediated disorders as well as some hematologic malignancies. Symptoms of hypomania, mania, depression, and psychosis are possible during medically indicated corticosteroid therapy and are dose related.[7]

Most patients treated with supraphysiologic doses of glucocorticosteroids will respond with an elevation of mood and a sense of well-being that is disproportionate to the state of their disease and sometimes mimicking a manic or hypomanic state.[2] Psychotic manifestations may also occur; for some patients, glucocorticoids induce depressive symptoms.

Depressive Disorders

Major Depressive Disorder with Irritable Mood

In some instances, the predominant mood in a patient with a major depressive disorder is not sadness, but rather irritability. Manifestations can include persistent anger, an exaggerated sense of irritation or frustration in response to minor annoyances, and a tendency to respond to events with angry outbursts or blaming others.[1] This presentation may be more common in children and adolescents.

> *Depressive symptoms need to be scrutinized for past, present, or future hypomanic, manic, or mixed symptoms to be differentiated from bipolar disorder.*

It can be difficult to differentiate this presentation of depression from a manic episode with irritable mood, from mixed episodes, or from mixed or dysphoric hypomania. The differential diagnosis requires a careful clinical evaluation to detect symptoms of mania (e.g., decreased need for sleep, increased energy, impulsivity) and differentiate them from those of irritability with depression. The individual's past history and family history are important for developing a full picture of the symptoms.

Dysthymic Disorder

Dysthymic disorder is commonly found in a primary care setting and can present in children, adolescents, and adults. It is characterized by depressed mood for most of the day, for more days than not, for at least two years.[1] Criteria may be met by either self-report or by history obtained from others. Patients must have at least two of the following neurovegetative symptoms:

- Poor appetite or overeating
- Insomnia or hypersomnia
- Low energy or fatigue
- Low self-esteem
- Poor concentration or difficulty making decisions
- Feelings of hopelessness

Depression symptoms may include irritability, pessimism, and low social involvement. Differentiation of dysthymic disorder from major depressive episode in a patient with bipolar disorder requires a history of mania or hypomania in the latter. In the absence of a history of mania/hypomania, a diagnosis of bipolar disorder cannot be made.

Schizophrenia and Schizoaffective Disorder

Schizoaffective disorder consists of symptoms of schizophrenia and major affective disorder (e.g., bipolar disorder, major depressive disorder). The DMS-IV (TR) diagnosis of schizoaffective disorder requires an uninterrupted period of illness characterized by active symptoms of schizophrenia plus concurrent manifestations of either a major depressive disorder, manic episode, or mixed episode (manic, depressive).[1] During the course of schizoaffective symptoms, the patient must also experience delusions or hallucinations for at least two weeks (**in the absence of prominent mood symptoms**). Lastly, mood symptoms should be present for a substantial portion of both the active and residual phases of the illness. Manic symptoms occur in the bipolar subtype of schizoaffective disorder, but the course of illness is distinguished by persistence of psychosis significantly beyond remission of mania.

The bipolar subtype of schizoaffective disorder differs from bipolar disorder in persistence of psychotic symptoms significantly beyond duration of mood episodes.

Differentiation of mood disorder from schizophrenia can be difficult. Psychotic manifestations may be present in patients with bipolar disorder and mood disturbances are common during all phases of schizophrenia. Depressive symptoms especially occur in patients with chronic psychotic disorders. To differentiate the two, it is important to carefully chart a longitudinal history of the symptoms. Psychotic manifestations of patients with bipolar disorder primarily manifest themselves during periods of mood instability while the total duration of mood symptoms is relatively brief in patients with schizophrenia. Since there are differences in therapy for the two disorders, it is important to establish a precise diagnosis.

If psychotic manifestations are present, do not assume that the patient has schizophrenia. While psychotic manifestations may be present in patients with bipolar disorder, affective symptoms are not a major enduring component of schizophrenia. The diagnosis of schizophrenia should be one of exclusion of psychotic mood disorders.

Attention Deficit Hyperactivity Disorder (ADHD)

Attention deficit hyperactivity disorder (ADHD) is character-ized by a persistent pattern of inattention and/or hyperactive-impulsivity that is more common and severe than that observed in other individuals at a comparable stage of development.[1] While typically considered a disorder predominantly of children, manifestations can persist into adulthood for about half of the individuals. Features of the disorder that may raise the possibility of bipolar illness include hyperactivity (as if "driven by a motor") and impulsivity. While these syndromic manifestations may be suggestive of mania, functional and social impairments of ADHD may con-tribute to depression.

> *ADHD is distinguished from bipolar disorder by absence of racing thoughts, decreased need for sleep, grandiosity, psychosis.*

For individuals with ADHD, manifestations are often chronic and mixed. In bipolar disorder, manifestations are cyclic and euphoric or mixed, though it should be noted that, in children, bipolar disorder may present as more persistent and less cyclic. Family history of affective illness needs to be considered when evaluating a patient for ADHD versus bipolar disorder. Symp-toms characteristic of mania (but not ADHD per se) include:

- Pressured speech
- Grandiosity or persistently elevated mood

- Decreased need for sleep
- Psychosis
- Racing thoughts

Impulse Control Disorders

Impulse control disorders consist of a group of conditions that share the essential feature of being unable to resist an impulse, drive, or temptation to perform an action potentially harmful to the person or others.[1] In most instances, an individual with an impulse control disorder experiences an increasing sense of tension or arousal before committing the act. Impulse control disorders include kleptomania, pyromania, intermittent explosive disorder, and pathological gambling.

During the event, affected individuals experience pleasure, gratification, or relief. However, following the impulsive act, individuals often feel drained, exhausted, and depressed. The similarity between impulse control and bipolar disorder rests in the excessive involvement in pleasurable activities that have a high potential for painful consequences in both. Importantly, however, in patients with bipolar disorder these activities are a component of mania or possibly hypomania.

Psychotic Disorder NOS

This is a residual diagnostic category for patients displaying brief (one day to one month) psychotic symptoms not better accounted for by another illness.

Differential Diagnostic Tools

To improve identification of patients with bipolar disorders, Hirschfeld et. al. developed a three-part Mood Disorder Questionnaire (MDQ).[8] Subsequently, in collaboration with Dr. Hirschfeld, Compact Clinicals has developed the MDQ-Expanded, with additional features.[9]

Mood Disorders Questionnaire (MDQ)

The MDQ screens for a history of symptoms of mania or hypomania and the degree of functional impairment produced by these symptoms (No problem; Minor problem; Moderate problem; Serious problem).

> *The MDQ identified 70 percent of patients with bipolar disorder and correctly screened 90 percent of those without the disorder.*

Researchers validated the MDQ as a screening tool based on responses gathered from five outpatient clinics primarily treating patients with mood disorders. In this study, a research professional, unaware of the MDQ results, conducted a telephone research diagnostic interview by using the bipolar module of the Structured Clinical Interview for DSM-IV. The instrument demonstrated 73 percent sensitivity and 90 percent specificity for bipolar illness, when ≥7 symptoms were endorsed as occurring simultaneously.

The MDQ has been subsequently validated by other investigators.[10] The sensitivity of the MDQ significantly decreases when used to screen the general population instead of outpatients with mood disorders.

A positive MDQ indicates a more in depth clinical interview is warranted.

MDQ-Expanded

A new version of the Mood Disorder Questionnaire (MDQ-Expanded) offers screening for:[9]

- Current symptoms of mania (instead of only past ones)
- Depression
- Alcohol abuse

Comorbidities in Patients with Bipolar Disorder

Relative to the general population, patients with bipolar disorder have higher lifetime prevalence rates for many medical and psychiatric illnesses, including; cardiovascular disease, cancer, obesity, type 2 diabetes mellitus, substance abuse, anxiety disorders, personality disorders, and eating disorders.

The presence of comorbidities can complicate the diagnosis and treatment of bipolar disorder by:

Chapter 7: Strategic Treatment Considerations for Bipolar Disorder addresses treatment strategies for comorbid medical conditions as well as those for anxiety disorders and substance use/abuse — the two most prevalent psychiatric disorders comorbid with bipolar disorder.

- Impairing functional outcomes

- Contributing to cyclic acceleration and more severe episodes over time

- Complicating treatment due to drug interaction or impaired organ function

- Requiring aggressive treatment of comorbidities to improve long-term outcomes.

Medical Comorbidity

The presence of a comorbid medical condition interacts with bipolar disorder because:

- Medical conditions can both exacerbate and be exacerbated by bipolar disorder.

- Treatments for medical conditions and for bipolar disorder can exacerbate one another.

For example, the increased risk for obesity and type 2 diabetes, which can be exacerbated by weight gain from some treatments of bipolar disorder, suggests that monitoring of body weight, calculation of body mass index (BMI), and education about sound diet, nutrition and exercise are important components of treatment.[11] (See chapter 7 for further discussion of this issue.)

Psychiatric Comorbidity

The most common psychiatric comorbidities are substance-related, anxiety, personality, and eating disorders. For the primary care physician, the common association of these psychiatric disorders with bipolar disorder has a number of practical implications:[12]

Clinicians should evaluate:

- Comorbidities

- Other psychiatric disorders that may present for the first time after the diagnosis of bipolar disorder

- Children and adolescents for other Axis I disorder diagnostic criteria that may not have had sufficient time to evolve at first presentation of symptoms

- Patients presenting with substance-related, anxiety, personality, impulse control, and eating disorders for symptoms diagnostic of a mood disorder

- Young people with a family history of mood disorders, including bipolar illness, with an early-onset anxiety, substance use, or eating disorder for a prodromal mood disorder including bipolar disorder

Illness prevalence and comorbidity with bipolar disorder are:

- Substance Use/Abuse — 44 to 61 percent[13, 14]

- Anxiety Disorders — 24 to 42 percent[12, 15]

- Personality Disorders — 30 percent general prevalence (comorbidity is debated due to symptom overlap)

- Eating Disorders — 0.5 to 3 percent

References

1. American Psychiatric Association, American Psychiatric Association Task Force on DSM-IV. *Diagnostic and statistical manual of mental disorders: DSM-IV-TR.* Washington, DC, American Psychiatric Association, 2000.

2. Goodman LS, Hardman JG, Limbird LE, Gilman AG. *Goodman & Gilman's the pharmacological basis of therapeutics.* New York, McGraw-Hill, 2001.

3. Zocchi A, Girlanda E, Varnier G, Sartori I, Zanetti L, Wildish GA, Lennon M, Mugnaini M, Heidbreder CA. Dopamine responsiveness to drugs of abuse: A shell-core investigation in the nucleus accumbens of the mouse. *Synapse.* 2003; 50(4):293-302.

4. Hibbs J, Perper J, Winek CL. An outbreak of designer drug—related deaths in Pennsylvania. *JAMA.* 1991; 265(8):1011-3.

5. Tomkins DM, Sellers EM. Addiction and the brain: the role of neurotransmitters in the cause and treatment of drug dependence. *Cmaj.* 2001; 164(6):817-21.

6. Buchanan JF, Brown CR. 'Designer drugs.' A problem in clinical toxicology. *Med Toxicol Adverse Drug Exp.* 1988; 3(1):1-17.

7. Brown ES, Suppes T. Mood symptoms during corticosteroid therapy: a review. *Harvard Review of Psychiatry.* 1998; 5(5):239-46.

8. Hirschfeld RM, Williams JB, Spitzer RL, Calabrese JR, Flynn L, Keck PE, Jr., Lewis L, McElroy SL, Post RM, Rapport DJ, Russell JM, Sachs GS, Zajecka J. Development and validation of a screening instrument for bipolar spectrum disorder: the Mood Disorder Questionnaire. *Am J Psychiatry.* 2000; 157(11):1873-5.

9. Hirschfeld, R. and Compact Clinicals (2005). Mood Disorder Questionnaire-Expanded. Kansas City, Missouri: Compact Clinicals.

10. Hirschfeld RM, Holzer C, Calabrese JR, Weissman M, Reed M, Davies M, Frye MA, Keck P, McElroy S, Lewis L, Tierce J, Wagner KD, Hazard E. Validity of the mood disorder questionnaire: a general population study. *Am J Psychiatry.* 2003; 160(1):178-80.

11. Citrome L, Jaffe A, Levine J, Allingham B, Robinson J. Relationship between antipsychotic medication treatment and new cases of diabetes among psychiatric inpatients, *Psychiatr. Serv.* 2004 Sep; 55(9):1006-13.

12. McElroy SL, Altshuler LL, Suppes T, Keck PE, Jr., Frye MA, Denicoff KD, Nolen WA, Kupka RW, Leverich GS, Rochussen JR, Rush AJ, Post RM. Axis I psychiatric comorbidity and its relationship to historical illness variables in 288 patients with bipolar disorder. *Am J Psychiatry.* 2001; 158(3):420-6.

13. Regier DA, Farmer ME, Rae DS, Locke BZ, Keith SJ, Judd LL, Goodwin FK. Comorbidity of mental disorders with alcohol and other drug abuse. Results from the Epidemiologic Catchment Area (ECA) Study. *JAMA.* 1990; 264(19):2511-8.

14. McElroy SL, Altshuler LL, Suppes T, Keck PE, Jr., Frye MA, Denicoff KD, Nolen WA, Kupka RW, Leverich GS, Rochussen JR, Rush AJ, Post RM. Axis I psychiatric comorbidity and its relationship to historical illness variables in 288 patients with bipolar disorder. *Am J Psychiatry.* 2001; 158(3):420-6.

15. Henry C, Van den Bulke D, Bellivier F, Etain B, Rouillon F, Leboyer M. Anxiety disorders in 318 bipolar patients: prevalence and impact on illness severity and response to mood stabilizer. *J Clin Psychiatry.* 2003; 64(3):331-5.

Chapter 6: Neurobiology & Neuropsychology of Bipolar Disorder

There are no experimental animal models to allow us to understand the neuroanatomical basis of bipolar disorder. As a result, current knowledge about the neurological basis of this illness comes from several kinds of indirect evidence:

- Neuroanatomical abnormalities
- Functional anormalities
- Drug effects that modulate neurotransmitter systems
- Neuropsychological studies on subjects with the illness
- Behavioral sensitization and kindling models

Chapter 6 at a Glance

Neuroanatomy

Neuropathological and magnetic resonance imaging (MRI) procedures have been used to study the structure of the central nervous system in patients with bipolar disorder. Fractal dimension (FD) MRI has been used to examine structural abnormalities at the microscopic level. This procedure utilizes changes in signal intensities between the hydrophilic (predominantly cellular gray matter) and the hydrophobic (myelin-rich white matter). In patients with bipolar disorder, studies of the cortical/subcortical interface demonstrate an increase in FD of the region that indicates an alteration in the ratio of gray to white matter.[1] Advantages of MRI include the ability to image both soft tissue and structure and function without using ionizing radiation.[2] However, several issues complicate interpretation of these studies:[3]

1. The recurrent nature of the illness and intercurrent periods of euthymia suggest that the disease has a dynamic neurophysiological and neurochemical as well as a contributing neuroanatomical basis.

2. Studies have reported conflicting results.

3. Changes in the brain may result from long-term pharmacotherapy rather than from the disease itself.

4. Few studies have been done on first-episode patients.

Neuroanatomical Abnormalities in Bipolar Disorder Patients

A variety of common structural abnormalities have been studied in the brains of patients with bipolar illness, including:

- White Matter Hyperintensities (WMH)

- Ventricular Enlargement or Sulcal Widening

- Limbic Structure Changes

- Frontal and Prefrontal Cortex (PFC) Abnormalities

- Cerebellum Atrophy
- Volume Enhancement

White Matter Hyperintensities (WMH)

The most consistently reported and studied abnormality is the presence of hyperintensities in the white matter. WMH reflect imaging findings associated with cerebrovascular disorders and aging, and are considered rare in healthy populations under the age of 40. Although the impact for clinical course and outcome is still unknown, a number of observations support the link between bipolar illness and WMH. In a study of 75 patients, Altshuler et. al. reported that patients with bipolar disorder showed no significant imaging differences in subcortical gray or deep matter when they were compared with controls.[4] However, patients with bipolar disorder had significantly more periventricular hyperintensities (bipolar I > bipolar II). A metaanalysis of pooled data from the literature reported that a bipolar I diagnosis, in particular, significantly increases the chance of finding this white matter abnormality. Recent reports have noted WMH differences are also significant in children and adolescents with early onset bipolar disorder compared to age-matched controls.[5, 6]

Ventricular Enlargement or Sulcal Widening

An indicator of cortical atrophy, CT scans illustrate that as many as one-fourth of patients with bipolar disorder have cortical or cerebellar atrophy.[3] Although sulcal widening can also been seen in patients with schizophrenia, widening of the cerebellar sulci seems to be more prominent in patients with bipolar illness.[7] Although ventricular enlargement occurs in patients with bipolar illness, it appears to be non-specific since it is also a common manifestation of schizophrenia. However, the degree of ventricular enlargement may relate to outcome. Kato et. al. reported that bipolar patients with psychotic features had significantly greater ventricular enlargement than those without.[8] However, results of ventricular enlargement are inconsistent, with some studies reporting significant differences.[2] More recent MRI research has focused on specific brain regions.[9]

Limbic Structure Changes

Since the limbic region is thought to be a central element in mood regulation, there have been extensive studies of limbic structures in patients with mood disorders. Changes in this region are subtle with little evidence of volume reduction. Studies suggest that there may be an increased volume in limbic system elements, such as the amygdala.[10–13] However, results vary across studies, and a recent study on hippocampal and amygdala volumes in adolescents with bipolar disorder found no volume increase relative to healthy controls.[14] Studies of the caudate have also demonstrated an increased volume, though no changes have been identified in other structures, such as the putamen and globus pallidus.[15] Vascular or mass lesions of the right cerebral hemisphere have been linked to changes in affect that may mimic similar symptoms of bipolar disorder. Neither MRI nor CT scans have demonstrated specific, right-hemispheric abnormalities in patients with bipolar disorder, though a recent pilot study found right-sided and gender-specific differences in the prefrontal cortex.[3, 16]

Frontal Cortex and Prefrontal Cortex (PFC) Abnormalities

Involved in stress-related autonomic and neuroendocrine responses among other functions, the PFC participates in reinforcing activities through mesolimbic dopaminergic circuitry. Drevet et. al. conducted a histopathological assessment of PFC tissue from in-patients with major depressive and bipolar disorders.[17] They reported that the PFC was selectively decreased in non-neuronal (glial) elements, suggesting that this alteration may be linked to clinical manifestations in patients with mood disorders. Studies are variable, though generally a decrease in gray matter assessed by MRI has been observed in prefrontal, frontal, and cingulate regions.[11, 18, 19] In some cases, differences between hemispheres have been noted, but these studies lacked consistent findings and large sample sizes.

Cerebellum Atrophy

While decreases in cerebellum size due to atrophy have been observed, it is difficult to interpret these findings due to potential confounds, including age, medical and substance use history, and course of illness history.[2]

Volume Enhancement

There is the increasing recognition that some medications used to treat psychiatric illness have neurotropic properties. Two recent studies found increased cerebral gray matter following relatively short periods of lithium treatment.[20, 21] Other studies are underway to understand these phenomena and to assess other medications for similar effects.

Functional Abnormalities in Bipolar Patients (fMRI, MRS, PET, SPECT)

Functional neuroimaging (fMRI) uses noninvasive techniques to detect changes in either of the following:[2, 22]

- The cerebral blood oxygen level
- The cellular metabolism that identifies areas of brain activation

In fMRI, as regional cellular activity increases in response to alterations in specific brain activities, blood flow to the region and oxygen extraction increase to meet tissue requirements. This increase creates an imbalance between oxygen supply and demand that results in an associated decrease in the concentration of deoxyhemoglobin in post-capillary venules draining the metabolically active site. By contrast, magnetic resonance spectroscopy (MRS) shows the amount of different chemicals in a given brain region.

Two additional functional imaging techniques using low amounts of radiation are:

- Positron emission tomography (PET)
- Single photon emission computed tomography (SPECT)

Both techniques utilize short, half-life radioisotopes to assess blood flow and glucose utilization, both viewed as indices of brain activity. Advances in PET and SPECT now allow detailed assessment of synaptic receptors, transporters, and certain key enzymes.

Functional MRI

Functional MRI combines conventional MRI resolution with fast imaging techniques to detect metabolism-associated alterations in the ratio of oxyhemoglobin to deoxyhemoglobin. Changes in the magnetic susceptibility can be used to identify regions of brain activation. Thus, decreases in deoxyhemoglobin are taken as a measure of brain activity.

Although fMRI studies in patients with bipolar disorder have produced varying results, cerebral blood flow alterations appear consistently across studies in symptomatic patients.

Studies of fMRI by definition utilize a task to assess brain function. To date, studies on emotional (happy/sad faces) and cognitive testing (e.g., a neurocognitive test, such as the Stroop Task) have used this powerful and direct test of location-specific brain activity. The potential to develop a circuit theory of emotion or define the "functional neuroanatomy" is advancing rapidly.[13, 23]

Two studies utilizing emotional stimuli found increased recruitment of subcortical regions, including the amygdala, thalamus, and globus pallidus in patients with bipolar disorder relative to the control group.[24, 25] One of these studies found decreased frontal activation as well.[24]

Recent studies using neurocognitive probes have observed complex state- and trait-dependent changes in the prefrontal cortex, supporting and extending earlier studies. New work from the Blumberg group reports:[26]

- Decreased ventral prefrontal cortex (VPFC) in patients with bipolar disorder currently hypomanic
- Increased left VPFC in depressed patients

Earlier studies found decreased activity on the left hemishere for depression and on the right for mania, but not all studies have supported this distinction. Other earlier work in depression suggested ventral regions were increased and dorsal regions decreased of the prefrontal cortex and anterior cingulate cortex, while mania was the reverse.[26]

Further studies on an adolescent population with bipolar disorder found increased activation of subcortical areas, including the putamen and the thalamus. Prefrontal abnormalities reported for adults with bipolar disorder were not observed, but developmental changes observed in healthy controls were not observed in adolescent patients with bipolar disorder. This age correlation may reflect a developing defect that is correlated positively with age in the PFC.[27]

These recent reviews indicate the dynamic nature of the MRI field and the potential to rapidly and significantly increase our understanding of brain function in health and illness.

Magnetic Resonance Spectroscopy (MRS)

MRI hardware and specialized software can be combined to evaluate various tissue metabolite concentrations in response to cortical activities. For example, increased concentrations of N-acetylaspartate (NAA) indicate neuronal and synaptic activity, while changes in high-energy, phosphate compounds reflect cerebral metabolism.

MRS typically uses H (hydrogen) or P (proton) MRS techniques, each allowing measurement of different brain chemicals.[2] Recent findings using this activated imaging include a metaanalysis assessing the relative ratio of compounds possibly related to membrane defects that are altered in patients with bipolar disorder relative to healthy controls.[28]

Other studies have found broad decreases in NAA and choline, as well as potential mitochrondrial defects in those with bipolar, all suggestive of neuronal dysfunction at a chemical level for patients with bipolar disorder.[29–31] Confirming that certain of these abnormalities may be trait related, another recent study in children with bipolar disorder (who had at least one parent with the disorder) found decreases in NAA and other compounds and an increase of myo-inositol in the frontal cortex compared to matched controls, suggestive of impairment in the basic phosphoinositide metabolism pathway.[32]

Positron Emission Tomography (PET)

Cognition is associated with changes in cerebral blood flow and an associated increase in glucose utilization. PET employs radioactive positron emitter isotopes incorporated into various metabolic substrates to:

- Localize areas of cerebral activation
- Evaluate metabolic activity
- Determine the location of neurotransmitters and associated receptor binding

For example, metabolic activity can be evaluated by the use of radioactive fluorodeoxyglucose. The radioactivity emitted by the labeled molecules is then measured by gamma-ray detectors and used to create an anatomic model of cerebral metabolism.

Functional imaging studies have found several types of changes in cerebral blood flow associated with unipolar and bipolar disorder, including:[33]

- Global reductions

- Bilateral decreases in the hypofrontal region

- Lower overall perfusion in the temporal lobes

One of the main findings in resting state studies appears to be decreased blood flow in the prefrontal cortex, anterior cingulate cortex, and caudate.[34] PET scans have identified the sub-genual prefrontal cortex and the anterior cingulate gyrus as areas of decreased glucose metabolism in patients with depression, both unipolar and bipolar.[35] The change in the caudate may also be a significant observation in view of the extensive connections between the caudate, prefrontal cortex, and amygdala: all structures known to be involved in affective processes.

Blumberg et. al. provide a summary of recent PET studies that focus more specifically on patients with bipolar disorder. They report:[36]

- Increased anterior cingulate and basal ganglia activity in resting PET scans during elevated mood states (in some cases hypomania, and in others, mania)

- Confirmatory increased activity in these same areas during mania versus euthymia, especially located in the left hemisphere

This report reviews earlier studies of somewhat different findings.[30] New studies are now examining brain activation during a task in different mood states and considering the possibility of predicting treatment response by premedication PET scan.[37, 38]

Single Proton Emission CT (SPECT)

Radioisotopes used for SPECT studies emit a single gamma ray rather than a positron. While lowering the spatial resolution due to a single gamma ray, the cost is also lower per scan than PET. Similar to PET, SPECT studies may be made of cerebral blood flow and radioligand binding. Results evaluating brain activity through changes in blood flow support:[2, 36, 39, 40]

- Decreased activity in depression.

- Increased anterior cingulate activity in mania.

- Increased temporal lobe and anterior cingulate activity in mania (These studies captured changes in brain perfusion either for a patient moving from euthymia to mania with lithium discontinuation or in rapid cycling patients experiencing different states where longitudinal studies were collected.)[29, 40]

In sum, we anticipate improved understanding of the functional neuroanatomy of patients with bipolar disorder in the next few years. Neuroimaging study goals include understanding brain function and dysregulation as well as improving treatments and management.[41]

Neurotransmitter Systems

As our understanding of bipolar disorder has evolved, we recognize that its clinical manifestations are, in part, a function of the interactions of the six, major neurotransmitter systems that regulate both mood and behavior. Additionally, information is evolving on the complex role of bioactive co-transmitters and secondary modulators of established neurotransmitters.

Because the variety of neurotransmitters are distributed throughout the central nervous system (CNS), drugs that impact one neurotransmitter may be particularly effective for treating one disorder but will also affect other brain areas. For example, the midbrain's dopamine receptors (involved in psychosis) are a site of action of classic or typical antipsychotics, which also act on the basal ganglia causing side effects.

Noradrenergic System

The noradrenergic system targets the thalamus, limbic structures, and cortex to modulate mood, sleep cycles, appetite, and cognition. Norepinephrine is synthesized from dopamine by the enzyme dopamine-b-hydroxylase. Once synthesized, it is stored in synaptic vesicles in noradrenergic neurons. Approximately one-half of noradrenergic neurons are located in the locus coeruleus. From there, they innervate the hypothalamus, basal forebrain, and spinal cord. They bind to the α_1, α_2 and β_2 receptors.

Dopaminergic System

Dopaminergic neurons of the substantia nigra project to the striatum and are involved in fine-tuning motor activities. Neurons of the dopaminergic mesolimbic pathways synapse on the nucleus accumbens and are implicated in reinforcement (e.g., in substances of abuse). Dopaminergic neurons in the hypothalamus also tonically inhibit the production and release of prolactin from the pituitary gland.

Abnormalities of dopaminergic neurotransmission are central elements in Parkinson's disease, schizophrenia, and psychosis. Extrapyramidal side effects of various antipsychotic drugs are the result of decreased dopaminergic function. Dopamine binds to the receptors of the D_1 and D_2 families.

The D_1 receptor family includes the D_1 and the D_5 receptors. Both are coupled with metabotropic G proteins. Binding of dopamine to receptors in the D_1 family leads to increased intracellular levels of cAMP through the medium of a stimulatory G protein (Gs). The D_2 receptor family includes D_2, D_3, and D_4 receptors. When bound to an inhibitory G protein (Gi), D_2 receptor family members decrease intracellular cAMP.

Serotonergic System

Projections of serotonergic neurons are involved in a number of brain functions (e.g., anxiety, regulation of mood, thoughts, aggression, appetite, sex drive). Modulation of serotonergic recep-

Newer generation psychotropics demonstrate mixed dopamine and serotonin receptor activity, perhaps accounting, in part, for their mood-stabilizing effects on bipolar illness.

tors and 5-HT reuptake is beneficial in a number of psychiatric disorders, including depression, anxiety, bipolar illness, obsessive compulsive disorder, and schizophrenia. Lower levels of serotonin have been found in postmortem studies of those who have committed suicide. Three receptors are currently identified $5\text{-}HT_{1\text{-}3}$.

The chemistry of the newer generation psychotropics (atypical antipsychotics), is an example of the likely role of the serotonergic pathways in psychotic disorders and bipolar illness. Unlike conventional antipsychotics, many of these drugs demonstrate mixed dopamine and serotonin receptor activity (i.e., dopamine-serotonin stabilization). Researchers hypothesize that this mixture could be responsible for drugs in this class improving both the positive and negative symptoms of schizophrenia, as well as their mood stabilizing properties for patients with bipolar disorder.

GABAergic System

Gamma-aminobutyric acid (GABA) is the major inhibitory neurotransmitter in the CNS Modulation of GABAergic transmissions is used therapeutically to treat seizure, anxiety, agitation, and insomnia with drugs, such as benzodiazepines and barbiturates. GABAergic excitation acts to dampen excitation in other neuronal systems. Enhancement of GABA activity is one of the roles of many antiepileptic agents. GABA A and B receptors have been identified.

Glutamatergic System

Glutamate, the most abundant amino acid in the CNS, is a major excitatory neurotransmitter for central neurons. For example, glutamate excess may be associated with seizures. Excessive activation of glutamate receptors can be neurotoxic and may lead to neuronal degeneration and death. One potential mechanism of action of lithium, anticonvulsants, and antipsychotic drugs is to protect neurons from potential glutamate-induced neurotoxicity. Glutamate binds to a number of ionotropic and metabotropic sites, including the NMDA (N-methyl-O-aspartate) and AMPA (alpha-amino-3-hydroxy-5-methylisoxazole propionate) receptors.

Cholinergic System

Within the CNS, acetylcholine plays a role in cognitive functioning, memory, sleep/wake cycles, and motor control. Acetylcholine is a major transmitter in the peripheral nervous system that acts at the neuromuscular junction, in autonomic ganglia, and at the synapse of parasympathetic post-ganglionic fibers. Acetylcholine binds to either muscarinic or nicotinic receptors.

Histaminergic System

Histamine functions as a neurotransmitter within the CNS. Stimulation of H_1 receptors increases wakefulness and inhibits appetite. Thus, researchers hypothesize that the blockade of histaminergic receptors by antipsychotic and other drugs may contribute to sedation and weight gain.

Proposed Role for Multiple Neurotransmitter Systems in Bipolar Disorder

The neurochemistry of bipolar disorder is complex. An example of this may be seen in the story of one neurotransmitter. GABA is the major inhibitory neurotransmitter. Increased GABA release at the synapse of inhibitory neurons can increase release of other neurotransmitters (e.g., be indirectly excitatory), while release of GABA into the synapse of excitatory neurons can inhibit neurotransmission. For example, research results indicate that:

- Patients with bipolar disorder (who were manic or euthymic) had significantly lower peripheral plasma levels of GABA than did controls.[42, 43]

- Initial levels of GABA predicted medication response.[44]

- More-complex trophic function of GABA exists in the developing brain and possibly in the mature brain.[45]

- There is an actual deficit of GABA in postmortem studies of those with major depressive disorder, bipolar disorder, and schizophrenia.[46]

DOPA decarboxylase (L-amino acid decarboxylase), which catalyzes the synthesis of dopamine, norepinephrine, and serotonin, is believed to have neuromodulating properties. Abnormalities of DOPA decarboxylase genes have been reported in patients with bipolar illness; this observation suggests that dopaminergic dysfunction may contribute to the pathogenesis of the disorder.[47] Acting through the mesolimbic dopaminergic circuitry, dopamine is involved in the reinforcing (reward) properties of a variety of behaviors, including substance abuse, recognition of affect (happy, sad), and (potentially) modulation of impulsive behaviors.

A number of neurotransmitter systems influence dopamine release, including serotonergic, noradrenergic, and cholinergic systems. Brain studies of patients with bipolar illness indicate that they have alterations in 5-HT_{1A}, 5-HT_{1B}, and 5-HT_{2A} mRNA.[48] Atypical antipsychotics used in the treatment of bipolar disorder and schizophrenia affect dopaminergic (D_1, D_2, D_3), serotonergic (5-HT_{1A}, 5-HT_{2A}), adrenergic (a_1, a_2), muscarinic (M_1), and histaminergic (H_1) pathways. These findings support dysregulation of the serotonergic system in patients with mood disorders.

One of the neurotransmitter systems that has been an increasing focus of research efforts is the glutamatergic system. This system, traditionally considered neuroexcitatory, is now also seen to be central in functions of neuronal plasticity and resilience.[49] Research is actively assessing if medications directly acting on this system, as well as other neurotrophic agents, may be future therapeutic targets.[50]

Secondary Messenger Systems and Bipolar Disorder

The importance of secondary messengers has been increasingly recognized in bipolar disorder and other psychiatric and medical conditions.[51] Secondary messengers accomplish a number of physiologic functions responsible for neuronal activity. For example, they can activate protein kinases (PK) that induce transcription factors and other modulators of neuronal function.

Studies have demonstrated that second messengers appear to play an important role in lithium's mood stabilizing properties. Lithium is an uncompetitive inhibitor of the enzymes that modulate inositol transport and hydrolysis. In addition, it plays a role in the activity of PKC isozymes and the expression of the major PKC substrate MARCKS (myristoylated alanine-rich C-kinase substrate). The extracellular, signal-regulated kinase (ERK) is a G-protein-linked second messenger. Alterations in the brain-derived neurotropic factor (BDNF)-ERK pathway can produce a variety of changes in behaviors.

In therapeutic paradigms, lithium and valproate vigorously "upregulate" the ERK pathway. Thus, one of the potential mechanisms for the mood-stabilizing properties of these two drugs in patients with mania is modulation of second messengers involved in the activity of this kinase.[52-54]

Receptors for the various neurotransmitter systems are classified as one of the following:

- **Ionotropic** — Following binding of a neurotransmitter (e.g., ACH, GABA, glutamate, or 5-HT) to its receptor, the complex modulates ligand-gated ion channels that mediate synaptic transmission. Alterations in ion channels affect the state of activity of the cell (e.g., excitatory or inhibitory) by allowing flow of ions across the cell membranes.

- **Metabotropic** — These receptors bind neurotransmitter and neuroactive substances (e.g., dopamine, 5-HT, norepinephrine, and endogenous opioids and cannabinoids). The receptors are coupled to G-proteins, trimeric structures composed of an a- (bound to GTP) and a b-g dimmer (interacts with the a-subunit bound to GTP in the inactive state). Binding of the agonist activates the G-protein leading to conversion of GTP to GDP and dissociation of the a- and b-g subunits. Both the a-monomer and the b-g dimmer can then interact with a second-messenger generating enzyme. This activates the target enzyme with generation of second messengers, such as cyclic adenosine monoplyophate (cAMP), inositol triphosphate (ITP), and diacylglycerol (DAG). The b-g subunit can also modulate the activity of ligand-gated Na+, Ca++, and K+ ion channels.

Cognitive defects in patients with bipolar disorder may be due to defects in the circuitry of the frontal cortex and basal ganglia that have been identified in functional imaging studies described earlier. This seems to be a reasonable proposal, given the role of subcortical nuclei in working memory, rule-based learning, and planning future actions. In addition, the memory and learning disturbances and impulsive behavior seen in patients with the disorder support a dysfunction of temporolimbic elements, which are also suggested in neuroimaging studies (see earlier section).

Neuropsychology

Patients with bipolar disorder can have significant and persistent neurocognitive defects. Outside of acute episodes, general intellectual function is largely preserved. There are no significant differences in cognitive function between patients with unipolar or bipolar depression.[55] While patients with bipolar disorder in remission can outperform stable patients with schizophrenia on most tests of neurocognitive function, this advantage disappears during times of acute illness.[55]

Patients tend to suffer from attentional abnormalities, impaired executive functioning, and memory problems.

- **Attentional Abnormalities** — In patients with symptomatic illness, attentional abnormalities (e.g., defects of sustained attention and inhibitory control) are present and may persist even in remission.

- **Impaired Executive Functioning** — Planning, abstract concept formation, and set shifting — all features of executive functioning — are impaired in symptomatic patients with the disorder. Importantly, the patient's performance on tests of executive functioning can be affected by the presence of residual symptoms; however, executive functioning may also be normal in fully recovered patients.[55] A number of recent studies in euthymic patients have found a degree of impairment across multiple domains.[56-58]

- **Memory Problems** — In euthymic subjects diagnosed with bipolar illness, verbal memory may be impaired in some patients, and visio-spatial memory deficits may also be present.

Behavioral Sensitization and Kindling Models in Bipolar Illness

Increased behavioral responses can occur from one of two processes:

1. **Behavioral sensitization models**, where repeating the same dose of psychomotor stimulant or agonist reinforces a behavior.

2. **Kindling models**, where repeating a sub-threshold electrical stimulus to the brain over a period of days becomes supra-threshold and causes epileptic seizures. Theoretically, kindling may account for a person's symptoms becoming more frequent and severe over time without an increase of the initial trigger. For

example, patients with epilepsy, who have repeated seizures, appear to be more likely to have further seizures over time and to become increasingly refractory to drug therapy.

In early onset bipolar disorder, the weight of environmental stressors in genetically predisposed subjects may be episode triggers, with later episodes requiring less environmental influence to precipitate an attack. However, recent research does not support this theory as fully explanatory of the cycle acceleration seen in some patients. but not others.[60, 61] These mechanisms might also partially explain the influence of some drugs on the course of bipolar disorder.[62] For example, the mood-stabilizing properties of antiepileptic drugs, such as carbamazepine, might be due to their anti-sensitization/anti-kindling activity on limbic neurons. In contrast, the mood-elevating properties of antidepressants might favor the developing of rapid cycling or cycle acceleration.[3] However, in the absence of understanding of bipolar disorder's biologic underpinnings, these theoretical processes remain provisional. If proven, the hypotheses behind these processes support the need for early and aggressive therapy.

References

1. Strakowski SM, Woods BT, Tohen M, Wilson DR, Douglass AW, Stoll AL. MRI subcortical signal hyperintensities in mania at first hospitalization. *Biol Psychiatry.* 1993; 33(3):204-6.

2. Stoll AL, Renshaw PF, Yurgelun-Todd DA, Cohen BM. Neuroimaging in bipolar disorder: what have we learned? *Biol Psychiatry.* 2000; 48:505-17.

3. Bearden CE, Hoffman KM, Cannon TD. The neuropsychology and neuro-anatomy of bipolar affective disorder: a critical review. *Bipolar Disord.* 2001; 3(3):106-50; discussion 151-3.

4. Altshuler LL, Curran JG, Hauser P, Mintz J, Denicoff K, Post R. T2 hyperintensi-ties in bipolar disorder: magnetic resonance imaging comparison and literature meta-analysis. *Am J Psychiatry.* 1995; 152(8):1139-44.

5. Lyoo IK, Lee HK, Jung JH, Noam GG, Renshaw PF. White matter hyperintensi-ties on magnetic resonance imaging of the brain in children with psychiatric disorders. *Compr Psychiatry.* 2002; 43:361-8.

6. Pillai JJ, Friedman L, Stuve TA, Trinidad S, Jesberger JA, Lewin JS, Findling RL, Swales TP, Schulz SC. Increased presence of white matter hyperintensities in adolescent patients with bipolar disorder. *Psychiatry Res.* 2002;114: 51-6.

7. Nasrallah HA, Jacoby CG, McCalley-Whitters M. Cerebellar atrophy in schizophrenia and mania. *Lancet.* 1981; 1(8229):1102.

8. Kato T, Shiori T, Murashita J, Hamakawa H, Inubushi T, Takahashi S. Phos-phorus-31 magnetic resonance spectroscopy and ventricular enlargement in bipolar disorder. *Psychiatry Res.* 1994; 55(1):41-50.

9. Brambilla P, Harenski K, Nicoletti MA, Mallinger AG, Frank E, Kupfer DJ, Keshavan MS, Soares JC. Anatomical MRI study of basal ganglia in bipolar disorder patients. *Psychiatry Res.* 2001; 106:65-80.

10. Altshuler LL, Bartzokis G, Grieder T, Curran J, Mintz J. Amygdala enlarge-ment in bipolar disorder and hippocampal reduction in schizophrenia: an MRI study demonstrating neuroanatomic specificity. *Arch Gen Psychiatry.* 1998; 55(7):663-4.

11. Strakowski SM, DelBello MP, Sax KW, Zimmerman ME, Shear PK, Hawkins JM, Larson ER. Brain magnetic resonance imaging of structural abnormalities in bipolar disorder. *Arch Gen Psychiatry.* 1999; 56(3):254-60.

12. Brambilla P, Harenski K, Nicoletti M, Sassi RB, Mallinger AG, Frank E, Kupfer DJ, Keshavan MS, Soares JC. MRI investigation of temporal lobe structures in bipolar patients. *J Psychiatr Res.* 2003; 37:287-95.

13. Strakowski SM, Adler CM, DelBello MP. Volumetric MRI studies of mood disorders: do they distinguish unipolar and bipolar disorder? *Bipolar Disord.* 2002; 4:80-8

14. Blumberg HP, Kaufman J, Martin A, Whiteman R, Zhang JH, Gore JC, Charney DS, Krystal JH, Peterson BS. Amygdala and hippocampal volumes

in adolescents and adults with bipolar disorder. *Arch Gen Psychiatry*. 2003a; 60:1201-8.

15. Aylward EH, Roberts-Twillie JV, Barta PE, Kumar AJ, Harris GJ, Geer M, Peyser CE, Pearlson GD. Basal ganglia volumes and white matter hyperintensities in patients with bipolar disorder. *Am J Psychiatry*. 1994; 151(5):687-93.

16. Sharma V, Menon R, Carr TJ, Densmore M, Mazmanian D, Williamson PC. An MRI study of subgenual prefrontal cortex in patients with familial and non-familial bipolar I disorder. *J Affect Disord*. 2003; 77:167-71.

17. Drevets WC, Ongur D, Price JL. Neuroimaging abnormalities in the subgenual prefrontal cortex: implications for the pathophysiology of familial mood disorders. *Mol Psychiatry*. 1998; 3(3):220-6, 190-1.

18. Lyoo IK, Kim MJ, Stoll AL, Demopulos CM, Parow AM, Dager SR, Friedman SD, Dunner DL, Renshaw PF: Frontal lobe gray matter density decreases in bipolar I disorder. *Biol Psychiatry*. 2004; 55:648-51.

19. Lopez-Larson MP, DelBello MP, Zimmerman ME, Schwiers ML, Strakowski SM. Regional prefrontal gray and white matter abnormalities in bipolar disorder. *Biol Psychiatry*. 2002; 52:93-100.

20. Moore GJ, Bebchuk JM, Wilds IB, Chen G, Manji HK, Menji HK. Lithium-induced increase in human brain grey matter. *Lancet* 2000. 356:1241-2.

21. Sassi RB, Nicoletti M, Brambilla P, Mallinger AG, Frank E, Kupfer DJ, Keshavan MS, Soares JC. Increased gray matter volume in lithium-treated bipolar disorder patients. *Neurosci Lett* 2002.329: 243-5.

22. Frank Y, Pavlakis SG. Brain imaging in neurobehavioral disorders. *Pediatr Neurol*. 2001; 25(4):278-87.

23. Drevets WC. Neuroimaging studies of mood disorders. *Biol Psychiatry*. 2000; 48:813-29.

24. Yurgelun-Todd DA, Gruber SA, Kanayama G, Killgore WD, Baird AA, Young AD. fMRI during affect discrimnation in bipolar affective disorder. *Bipolar Disord*. 2000; 2:237-48.

25. Malhi GS, Lagopoulos J, Ward PB, Kumari V, Mitchell PB, Parker GB, Ivanovski B, Sachdev P. Cognitive generation of affect in bipolar depression: an fMRI study. *Eur J Neurosci*. 2004; 19:741-54.

26. Blumberg HP, Leung HC, Skudlarski P, Lacadie CM, Fredericks CA, Harris BC, Charney DS, Gore JC, Krystal JH, Peterson BS. A functional magnetic resonance imaging study of bipolar disorder: state- and trait-related dysfunction in ventral prefrontal cortices. *Arch Gen Psychiatry*. 2003b; 60:601-9.

27. Blumberg HP, Martin A, Kaufman J, Leung HC, Skudlarski P, Lacadie C, Fulbright RK, Gore JC, Charney DS, Krystal JH, Peterson BS. Frontostriatal abnormalities in adolescents with bipolar disorder: preliminary observations from functional MRI. *Am J Psychiatry*. 2003c; 160: 1345-7.

28. Yildiz A, Sachs GS, Dorer DJ, Renshaw PF. 31P Nuclear magnetic resonance spectroscopy findings in bipolar illness: a meta-analysis. *Psychiatry Res*. 2001; 106:181-91.

29. Cecil KM, DelBello MP, Morey R, Strakowski SM. Frontal lobe differences in bipolar disorder as determined by proton MR spectroscopy. *Bipolar Disord.* 2002; 4(6):357-65.

30. Lyoo IK, Demopulos CM, Hirashima F, Ahn KH, Renshaw PF. Oral choline decreases brain purine levels in lithium-treated subjects with rapid-cycling bipolar disorder: a double-blind trial using proton and lithium magnetic resonance spectroscopy. *Bipolar Disord.* 2003; 5:300-6.

31. Soares JC. Contributions from brain imaging to the elucidation of pathophysiology of bipolar disorder. *Int J Neuropsychopharmacol.* 2003; 6:171-80.

32. Cecil KM, DelBello MP, Sellars MC, Strakowski SM. Proton magnetic resonance spectroscopy of the frontal lobe and cerebellar vermis in children with a mood disorder and a familial risk for bipolar disorders. *J Child Adolesc Psychopharmacol.* 2003; 13(4):545-55.

33. Soares JC, Mann JJ. The functional neuroanatomy of mood disorders. *J Psychiatr Res.* 1997; 31:393-432.

34. Kennedy SH, Javanmard M, Vaccarino FJ. A review of functional neuroimaging in mood disorders: positron emission tomography and depression. *Can J Psychiatry.* 1997; 42(5):467-75.

35. Drevets WC, Price JL, Simpson JR, Jr., Todd RD, Reich T, Vannier M, Raichle ME. Subgenual prefrontal cortex abnormalities in mood disorders. *Nature.* 1997; 386(6627):824-7.

36. Blumberg HP, Stern E, Martinez D, Ricketts S, de Asis J, White T, Epstein J, McBride PA, Eidelberg D, Kocsis JH, Silbersweig DA. Increased anterior cingulate and caudate activity in bipolar mania. *Biol Psychiatry.* 2000; 48:1045-52.

37. Rubinsztein JS, Fletcher PC, Rogers RD, Ho LW, Aigbirhio FI, Paykel ES, Robbins TW, Sahakian DJ. Decision-making in mania: a PET study. *Brain.* 2001; 124:2550-63.

38. Ketter TA, Kimbrell TA, George MS, Willis MW, Benson BE, Danielson A, Frye MA, Herscovitch P, Post RM. Baseline cerebral hypermetabolism associated with carbamazepine response, and hypometabolism with nimodipine response in mood disorders. *Biol Psychiatry.* 1999; 46:1364-74.

39. Gyulai L, Alavi A, Broich K, Reilley J, Ball WB, Whybrow PC. I-123 iofetamine single-photon computed emission tomography in rapid cycling bipolar disorder: a clinical study. *Biol Psychiatry.* 1997; 41:152-61.

40. Goodwin GM, Cavanagh JT, Glabus MF, Kehoe RF, O'Carroll RE, Ebmeier KP. Uptake of 99mTc-exametazime shown by single photon emission computed tomography before and after lithium withdrawal in bipolar patients: associations with mania. *Br J Psychiatry.* 1997; 170:426-30.

41. Benabarre A, Vieta E, Martín F, Lomeña F, Yatham L. Functional neuroimaging abnormalities in bipolar disorders: SPECT and PET-FDG studies. *Bipolar Disord.* 2003; 2:57-66.

42. Petty F. GABA and mood disorders: a brief review and hypothesis. *J Affect Disord.* 1995;34:275-281.

43. Petty F, Kramer GL, Fulton M, Moeller FG, Rush AJ. Low plasma GABA is a trait-like marker for bipolar illness. *Neuropsychopharmacology*. 1993; 9:125-32.

44. Petty F, Rush AJ, Davis JM, Calabrese JR, Kimmel SE, Kramer GL, et al. Plasma GABA predicts acute response to divalproex in mania. *Biol Psychiatry*. 1996; 39:278-84.

45. Owens DF, Kriegstein AR. Is there more to GABA than synaptic inhibition? *Nat Rev Neurosci*. 2002; 3:715-27.

46. Cotter D, Landau S, Beasley C, Stevenson R, Chana G, MacMillan L, et al. The density and spatial distribution of GABAergic neurons, labelled using calcium binding proteins, in the anterior cingulate cortex in major depressive disorder, bipolar disorder, and schizophrenia. *Biol Psychiatry*. 2002; 51:377-86.

47. Borglum AD, Kirov G, Craddock N, Mors O, Muir W, Murray V, McKee I, Collier DA, Ewald H, Owen MJ, Blackwood D, Kruse TA. Possible parent-of-origin effect of Dopa decarboxylase in susceptibility to bipolar affective disorder. *Am J Med Genet*. 2003; 117B:18-22.

48. Lopez-Figueroa AL, Norton CS, Lopez-Figueroa MO, Armellini-Dodel D, Burke S, Akil H, Lopez JF, Watson SJ. Serotonin 5-HT(1A), 5-HT(1B), and 5-HT(2A) receptor mRNA expression in subjects with major depression, bipolar disorder, and schizophrenia. *Biol Psychiatry*. 2004; 55(3):225-33.

49. Zarate CA, Jr., Du J, Quiroz J, Gray NA, Denicoff KD, Singh J, Charney DS, Manji HK. Regulation of cellular plasticity cascades in the pathophysiology and treatment of mood disorders: role of the glutamatergic system. *Ann N Y Acad Sci*. 2003; 1003:273-91.

50. Manji HK, Quiroz JA, Sporn J, Payne JL, Denicoff K, Gray A, Zarate CA, Jr., Charney DS. Enhancing neuronal plasticity and cellular resilience to develop novel, improved therapeutics for difficult-to-treat depression. *Biol Psychiatry*. 2003; 53:707-42.

51. Gould TD, Manji HK. Signaling networks in the pathophysiology and treatment of mood disorders. *J Psychosom Res*. 2002; 53:687-97.

52. Lenox RH, Wang L. Molecular basis of lithium action: integration of lithium-responsive signaling and gene expression networks. *Mol Psychiatry*. 2003; 8:135-44.

53. Lenox RH, Hahn CG. Overview of the mechanism of action of lithium in the brain: fifty-year update. *J Clin Psychiatry*. 2000; 61 Suppl 9:5-15.

54. Manji HK, Lenox RH. The nature of bipolar disorder. *J Clin Psychiatry*. 2000; 61 Supp 13:42-57.

55. Quraishi S, Frangou S. Neuropsychology of bipolar disorder: a review. *J Affect Disord*. 2002; 72(3):209-26.

56. Fleck DE, Shear PK, Zimmerman ME, Getz GE, Corey KB, Jak A, Lebowitz BK, Strakowski SM. Verbal memory in mania: effects of clinical state and task requirements. *Bipolar Disord*. 2003; 5:375-80.

57. Martinez-Aran A, Vieta E, Reinares M, Colom F, Torrent C, Sanchez-Moreno J, Benabarre A, Goikolea JM, Comes M, Salamero M. Cognitive function across manic or hypomanic, depressed, and euthymic states in bipolar disorder. *Am J Psychiatry*. 2004; 161:262-70.

58. Zalla T, Joyce C, Szoke A, Schurhoff F, Pillon B, Komano O, Perez-Diaz F, Bellivier F, Alter C, Dubois B, Rouillon F, Houde O, Leboyer M. Executive dysfunctions as potential markers of familial vulnerability to bipolar disorder and schizophrenia. *Psychiatry Res*. 2004; 121:207-17.

59. Junque C, Pujol J, Vendrell P, Bruna O, Jodar M, Ribas JC, Vinas J, Capdevila A, Marti-Vilalta JL. Leuko-araiosis on magnetic resonance imaging and speed of mental processing. *Arch Neurol*. 1990; 47(2):151-6.

60. Hlastala SA, Frank E, Kowalski J, Sherrill JT, Tu XM, Anderson B, Kupfer DJ. Stressful life events, bipolar disorder, and the "kindling model". *J Abnorm Psychol*. 2000; 109:777-86.

61. Suppes T, Leverich GS, Keck PE, Nolen WA, Denicoff KD, Altshuler LL, McElroy SL, Rush AJ, Kupka R, Frye MA, Bickel M, Post RM. The Stanley Foundation Bipolar Treatment Outcome Network. II. Demographics and illness characteristics of the first 261 patients. *J Affect Disord*. 2001; 67:45-59

62. Post RM, Denicoff KD, Frye MA, Dunn RT, Leverich GS, Osuch E, Speer A. A history of the use of anticonvulsants as mood stabilizers in the last two decades of the 20th century. *Neuropsychobiology*. 1998; 38:152-66.

Chapter 7: Strategic Treatment Considerations for Bipolar Disorder

This chapter provides an introduction to bipolar disorder treatment strategies, including general treatment considerations and recommendations for:

- Pharmacological therapy and mitigating factors that may impact this approach

- Psychosocial therapy

- Electroconvulsive therapy

The balance of the book covers both pharmacological and psychosocial treatments in detail.

Chapter 7 at a Glance

Bipolar disorder is a lifetime illness and should be treated like any other recurrent condition. In general, the goals of treatment of bipolar disorder are to produce symptomatic remission, restoration of full psychosocial functioning, and prevention of relapses.

Chapters 8–10 review specific medication treatment options for mania, depression, and maintenance therapy. Chapter 11 reviews psychosocial treatments as well as efficacy studies.

In addition, psychosocial interventions are important treatment components that educate the patient about the illness, stress the importance of treatment adherence, identify potential stressors, and recognize and react to prodromal manifestations.

Pharmacological Treatment Strategies

Treatment should be conducted as a therapeutic alliance between the patient and clinician, with both parties identifying mild changes in mood or behavior that indicate prodromal manifestations, recognizing new episodes, instituting steps to optimize therapy, and managing adverse events.

During the early phase of treatment, careful monitoring is important to maximize pharmacotherapy and prevent patients from harming themselves or others. This is particularly important in mania — a mood state that may limit patients' insight into their behavior. The majority of attempted and completed suicides occur during depressive or mixed episodes.[1, 2]

The Texas Medication Algorithm Project (TMAP)

The Texas Medication Algorithm Project (TMAP) is a project that evaluated the clinical and economic impact of treatment guidelines for major psychiatric illnesses treated in the Texas Department of Mental Health and Mental Retardation system.[3] This project now continues as the Texas Implementation of Medication Algorithms (TIMA).

Treatment Algorithms

In 2002, the consensus of the conferees was subsequently condensed into a set of distinct algorithms for the treatment of bipolar I disorder (see figure 7.1 on page 7-7, for the algorithm for mania/hypomania and figure 7.2 on page 7-12, for the algorithm for depression). Treatment options in the algorithms are based upon evidence from the literature available at the time of the conference and expert consensus. Recommendations are divided into stages. In general, recommendations for the earlier stages are less complicated than those that follow and take into consideration the balance of efficacy, safety, and tolerability.

General Principles of the TIMA Strategy

The TIMA approach general principles include optimizing symptomatic remission with full return of psychosocial functioning and preventing relapses and recurrences.[3] The authors of the TIMA guidelines stress several important caveats to guide clinicians when treating patients with bipolar disorder (see table 7-1 below and on the next page).

Table 7-1. Important Strategic Treatment Considerations[3]

▲ Patients should be treated by the core algorithm.

▲ The algorithm focuses on the treatment of core symptoms.

▲ The most well-tolerated form of a given medication is recommended.

▲ Adjunctive medications are not described but may be required for comorbid conditions or symptoms such as anxiety.

▲ Treatment decisions progress through stages if there is an inadequate response to treatment or medication intolerance.

   ◆ Early stages include monotherapy with widely used medications.

   ◆ Later stages involve more complex medication

combinations with an attendant greater risk of side effects and monitoring requirements.

▲ **Medication changes should be made using an overlap-and-taper strategy unless medical necessity requires abrupt discontinuation.**

▲ **Severely ill patients should be evaluated more often (e.g., weekly) than patients who are less ill.**

▲ **All treatment decisions should be based on physician judgment and patient treatment history.**

▲ **A single week's improvements may not represent a stable drug effect.**

◆ After a clinical plateau is reached, patients should then be evaluated for at least two weeks until clinical stability is confirmed.

◆ If the patient is stable during the evaluation period, the clinician can assume that the response is stable and can start the patient on the continuation phase of treatment.

▲ **During the continuation phase of treatment:**

◆ See the patient monthly for the first three months.

◆ Thereafter, see patient at two- to three-month intervals.

Extracted from Suppes T et. al.. Report of the Texas Consensus Conference panel on medication treatment in bipolar disorder 2000. *J Clin Psychiatry* 2002;63:288-299.

Concept of Mood Stabilizers

The TIMA core algorithm for bipolar I disorder mania or hypomania and depression call for initial treatment with a mood stabilizer.

Lithium was the first "mood stabilizer." The term was created to describe lithium's combined antimanic and antidepressant activity.[4] Since that time, the term has been employed to describe psychotropic drugs that reduce vulnerability to subsequent episodes of mania or depression but do not exacerbate the current episodes or maintenance phase of therapy.[5] Today, in addition to lithium, the term mood stabilizer is applied to certain antiepileptic and atypical antipsychotic drugs. Debate continues as to the most appropriate definition of mood stabilizer. The classic definition is to improve both phases of the illness without worsening either phase and to be effective in prevention of new episodes.

According to the Expert Consensus Treatment Guidelines, to be classified as a mood stabilizer, a drug must:[6]

- Show efficacy in the treatment of acute mania and/or depression

- Provide effective prophylaxis for subsequent manic or depressive episodes

- Not worsen mood symptoms or acute episodes

- Not increase the likelihood of an affective switch or cycling

The American Psychiatric Association (APA) has developed general treatment recommendations for patients with bipolar disorder.[7] The recommendations for treatment throughout this chapter are a compilation of TIMA and APA guidelines, unless otherwise noted.[2, 7]

General Treatment Recommendations for Mania

The primary goals of therapy with antimanic agents (see chapter 8) are to rapidly control symptoms such as agitation, impulsivity, and aggression so that the patient can return to a normal level of functioning. Guidelines for selecting antimanic therapy include the severity of the patient's illness, the presence or absence of psychotic manifestations, and rapid cycling.

Treatment Algorithm for Mania

The strategy algorithm for treatment of mania/hypomania (figure 7.1 on page 7-7), as developed by the Texas Implementation of Medication Algorithms, describes these seven stages of therapy:

1. **Monotherapy with a mood stabilizer** — In patients who demonstrate a partial response to optimum levels of a single mood stabilizer, the options include adding a second agent or switching to another drug. However, patients who cannot tolerate a single agent should be switched to another drug.

2. **Combination therapy** — Standard care in most patients with bipolar mania. If the choice is between carbamazepine and oxcarbazepine, the latter is generally selected because of its more favorable tolerability profile. However, these are viewed as different drugs, and the data is more extensive for carbamazepine, particularly the long-acting formulation.

3. **Also combination therapy, generally substituting one of the two drugs for another agent** — If control of the illness is not achieved, advance to the next stage.

4. **Substitution of an atypical antipsychotic for one of the previous two medications** — Atypical antipsychotics can be added earlier if the patient has psychotic manifestations.

5. **"Triple" therapy** — Adds an atypical antipsychotic to Stage 4 combination therapy.

6. **Electroconvulsive therapy (ECT) or Clozapine** — Approach used at this point in patients with mania (late in the process due to safety, tolerability, and patient acceptance issues).

7. **Other therapies** — Utilizes other therapies only after stages one through six.

Since this medication algorithm was developed in 2000, several atypical antipsychotics have received FDA approval for bipolar mania and are now often used as first- and second-line agents. The inclusion of olanzapine as a first-line agent was based on completed, well-controlled trials in 2000. The authors anticipate that updates of these algorithms will include all atypical

Figure 7.1. Algorithm for Treatment of Mania/
Hypomania in Patients with Bipolar Disorder[3]

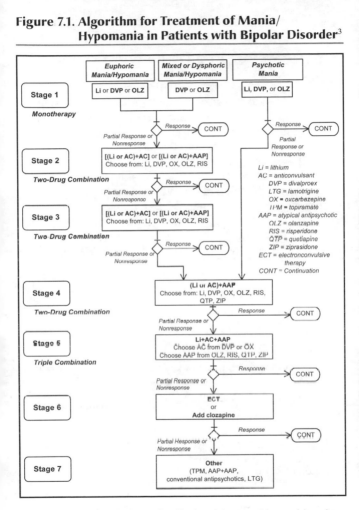

* Based on new FDA indications and applications, it is reasonable to anticipate future algorithms including newer atypical antipsychotics (e.g., risperidone, quetiapine, and others) at earlier stages.

(Public domain image from: Suppes T et al. Report of the Texas Consensus Conference panel on medication treatment in bipolar disorder 2000. *J Clin Psychiatr.* 2002;63:288-299.)

antipsychotics with good efficacy data (i.e., risperidone, quetiapine, ziprasidone, and aripiprazole).

> *Antimanic agents are reviewed in detail in chapter 8.*

Lithium, divalproex (valproate), and atypical antipsychotics are specified as first-line antimanic agents.[3] Lithium is not usually a first choice as monotherapy in patients with mixed symptoms (depression plus hypomania/mania symptoms) since patients with that presentation respond less well to it as a single agent. The divalproex form of valproate is usually recommended because of its more favorable side effect profile and tolerability. While olanzapine is listed as monotherapy for acute mania, the drug's adverse event profile and that of the other atypical antipsychotics should be considered before it or a member of this class is selected as first-line therapy. However, these agents now have FDA approval for use in acute mania.

Treatment Recommendations for Initial Approach to Therapy

- For patients with acute mania or mixed episodes, treatment should consist of either lithium or valproate combined with an atypical antipsychotic.

- For patients who are less severely ill (e.g., hypomania), monotherapy may be indicated.

- For patients with mixed episodes, valproate or atypical antipsychotics may be superior to lithium.

- If an antipsychotic must be administered, atypical antipsychotics are preferred because of their superior side effect profile.

- Antidepressants should be discontinued during treatment of acute mania.

- As the patient improves, psychosocial therapy should be combined with pharmacotherapy.

Treatment Recommendations for Breakthrough Episodes

- If patients presenting with acute mania or a mixed episode are currently receiving pharmacotherapy with a mood stabilizer, the first step should be to optimize current therapy.[7] Therefore, drug levels, when applicable, should be drawn at the time of presentation.

- If drug levels are within the therapeutic range, the dose may be increased to bring levels up to maximum dosage.

- If the patient is on monotherapy and has therapeutic drug levels, an atypical antipsychotic may be considered.

- Antipsychotics are also indicated when psychotic manifestations are present.

- Short-term treatment with a benzodiazepine can be used to decrease agitation, anxiety, and insomnia.

Treatment Recommendations for Inadequate Response to Initial Therapy

- Symptoms should be diminished within 10 to 14 days of therapy with optimized doses of first-line medications.[7]

- If treatment fails, alternative medications such as carbamazepine or an atypical antipsychotic may be added.

- It is important to confirm the diagnosis and ensure the clinical symptoms are not primarily due to a medical disorder or drug/alcohol substance use.

- If the current regimen already includes an atypical antipsychotic, the response may be improved if an alternate drug is substituted. For example, clozapine may be particularly effective in this situation for treatment-resistant patients.

- Electroconvulsive therapy (ECT) may be preferred for certain types of patients:

  — The severely ill

  — Those resistant to pharmacotherapy

  — Those with mixed episodes

  — The female patient with mania who is also pregnant

  — After consultation with a psychiatrist, those that preferentially select ECT

General Treatment Considerations for Acute Bipolar Depression

Guidelines for selecting antidepressant therapy include the severity of the patient's illness, the presence or absence of psychotic manifestations, and rapid cycling.

In general, combination therapy may be more effective than monotherapy in patients with more severe depression.

Treatment Algorithm for Acute Depression

The strategy algorithm for depression, as developed by the Texas Implementation of Medication Algorithms (TIMA), describes these six stages of therapy.[3]

1. **Monotherapy with a mood stabilizer** — Initiating or optimizing mood stabilizer therapy

2. **Combination therapy** — Adding medication to address major depressive symptom severity

3. **Switching antidepressant or different combination therapy** — Switching to a different antidepressant, adding venlafaxine or nefazodone, or adding a second antidepressant or lamotrigine

4. **Double antidepressant therapy** — Combining two antidepressant drugs, each from a different class (e.g., SSRI plus venlafaxine or bupropion) with mania treatment (drug interaction risk requires careful monitoring)

5. **MAOI/atypical antipsychotic therapy** — Utilizing an MAOI or adding an atypical antipsychotic when symptoms are refractory

Guidelines for selecting particular medications for an individual patient include:
- *Reported efficacy of the agent(s)*
- *Tolerability of side effects*
- *Potential drug interactions*
- *Side-effect profile*

6. **Other treatments** — Exploring remaining therapeutic options (e.g., electroconvulsive therapy, investigational compounds, tricyclic antidepressants)

(See Figure 7.2. Algorithm for Treatment of Depression in Patients with Bipolar I Disorder on page 7-12.)

The consensus recommendation of the TIMA was to treat depression in conjunction with mania/hypomania if symptoms of depression are sufficiently severe to warrant therapy.[3] Several issues complicate the decision to administer antidepressants, however. **Since antidepressant monotherapy can induce manic symptoms, drugs of this type must be administered only to depressed patients with bipolar I disorder who are also being treated with a mood stabilizer.** Furthermore, in a patient with apparent depression, depression must be carefully differentiated from dysphoric mania/hypomania or mixed symptoms and other more complicated states, since antidepressant monotherapy may simply unmask the mania. **Since the development of the TIMA algorithm, new data have emerged regarding olanzapine, olanzapine-fluoxetine combination, and quetiapine in the acute treatment of bipolar I depression.**

Figure 7.2. Algorithm for Treatment of Depression in Patients with Bipolar Disorder[3]*

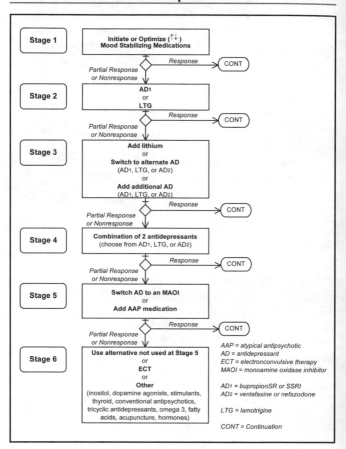

* To be used in conjunction with the primary treatment algorithm for mania/hypomania.

(Public Domain Image from: Suppes T et al. Report of the Texas Consensus Conference panel on medication treatment in bipolar disorder 2000. *J Clin Psychiatr.* 2002;63:288-299.)

Recommendations for Initial Approach to Therapy

The selection of initial therapy for the patient with acute bipolar depression should be based upon the presenting manifestations. In addition, patient preferences should be considered whenever possible.

- Combination therapy may be more effective than monotherapy in patients with more severe illness.

- Psychotic manifestations are an indication to add an antipsychotic to the regimen.

- When a patient presenting with an acute depressive episode gives a history of one or more prior untreated hypomanic or manic episodes, he or she should be treated with a mood stabilizer.

- Antidepressant monotherapy is contraindicated in bipolar I disorder, for reasons detailed above.

- Lithium or lamotrigine are reasonable initial therapeutic options.

- Certain atypical antipsychotics and olanzapine-fluoxetine combination are also therapeutic options.

- If the episode is particularly severe, lithium and antidepressant combination therapy is a prudent alternative [7]

- Electroconvulsive therapy (ECT) is a reasonable option for certain types of patients:

   − Those who are pregnant and severely depressed

   − When the risk of suicide is high.

   − If the patient has life-threatening unwillingness to eat, drink, or loss of vitality.

- After pharmacotherapy has been initiated, combination interpersonal therapy, cognitive behavioral therapy, or psychotherapy may be useful.

Treatment Recommendations for Breakthrough Episodes

- Optimizing medical therapy is the first step in a patient with acute bipolar depression who experiences one or more breakthrough episodes while being treated with one or more drugs.

- Serum drug levels should be obtained when appropriate (e.g., when treatment involves lithium).

- If the patient is on mood stabilizer monotherapy and drug levels are within the targeted range, an antidepressant should be added to the regimen. Reasonable agents include bupropion or paroxetine among other agents.

- If treatment already includes both a mood stabilizer and an antidepressant and drug levels are not within the therapeutic range, the doses should be increased.

- If levels are already within target range, doses should be increased until therapeutic drug concentrations are within the upper portion of the therapeutic range.

Treatment Recommendations for Inadequate Response to Initial Therapy

- If a patient treated with combination therapy fails to show an adequate response and has therapeutic drug levels within the targeted range, several additional steps can be considered.[7]

- The first step is to review the diagnosis and ensure that the depressive manifestations are not secondary to a general medical disorder or drug/alcohol use.

- Subsequently, one of the newer antidepressants (e.g., venlafaxine) or a monoamine oxidase inhibitor (MAOI) (e.g., tranylcypromine) can be added to the regimen.

- Importantly, MAOI therapy should be used cautiously because of the risk of severe hypertension due to dietary and drug interactions.

- If psychotic features are present, adjuvant antipsychotic therapy should be instituted.

- ECT should be considered when the patient is catatonic, fails to respond to any of the above measures, has psychotic features, or is suicidal.

Treatment Recommendations for Rapid Cycling

- Since rapid cycling may be due to or exacerbated by an associated general medical disorder such as hypothyroidism or substance use, a detailed history (including medications and drugs) should be obtained.

- Appropriate laboratory studies should also be obtained.

- Patients whose initial presentation includes rapid cycling should be treated with lithium, valproate, an atypical antipsychotic, or lamotrigine.

- If the bipolar nature of the process was unrecognized until the onset of cycling and the patient is being treated with antidepressant monotherapy, lithium, valproate, or lamotrigine should be added to the regimen and the dose of antidepressant tapered and discontinued, if possible.

- If, on the other hand, rapid cycling appears while the patient is being treated with a mood stabilizer and an antidepressant, combination regimens, possibly including an atypical antipsychotic, should be considered as well as tapering the antidepressant, if possible.

General Treatment Considerations for Maintenance Pharmacotherapy

Important considerations when selecting specific maintenance therapy for patients with bipolar disorder include severity of illness, presence of rapid cycling and/or psychosis, and reasonable patient preferences.

Maintenance therapy is indicated for patients with bipolar disorder following an episode of mania or depression.[3, 5, 7] Although studies are limited, it is also reasonable to institute maintenance therapy in patients with bipolar II disorder as the overall course, severity, and functional impacts are substantial.[1]

Therapy goals are to prevent relapse and recurrence of manic/hypomanic and major depressive episodes. Maintenance therapy should also reduce the likelihood that the patient will experience sub-syndromal symptoms. Appropriate maintenance therapy should improve functional outcomes and decrease suicide risk, frequency of cycling, and mood instability.

Maintenance Treatment Recommendations

- Since response to therapy of the acute episode documents a drug's primary efficacy, maintenance therapy usually includes the medications that led to remission from the last episode.

- Mood stabilizer therapy with lithium, valproate, lamotrigine, olanzapine, and clozapine has proven effective as maintenance therapy for bipolar I disorder.[7]

- Carbamazepine or oxcarbazepine are possible alternative medications.

- Although evidence is limited on the role of some atypical antipsychotics as maintenance therapy, reports suggest that patients treated with a mood stabilizer plus an atypical antipsychotic have a lower risk of relapse if the combination is continued as maintenance treatment.

- For patients who require ECT during an acute episode, it should be considered for maintenance therapy.

Treatment Recommendations for
Managing Patients Who Fail to Respond

- If the patient continues to experience breakthrough symptoms or mood instability, the first step should be to obtain drug levels and ensure that they are within the therapeutic range.

- If levels are low- to mid-range and side effects are minimal, the dose of the maintenance drug can be increased to achieve a level at the higher end of the therapeutic range.

- If the patient fails to respond to this approach, the clinician can supplement the mood stabilizer with a second maintenance agent.

- At this time, data are insufficient to make a definitive recommendation. However, the efficacy of lithium and lamotrigine at preventing recurrent manic and depressive episodes, respectively, suggest that this combination is a reasonable alternative.

Medication Efficacy

Key medications used for treating bipolar disorder have been studied extensively in recent clinical trials. On the next page, Table 7-2. Bipolar Disorder: Summary of Efficacy Evidence from Randomized Controlled Trials (RCTs) compares results by drug for treating mania, depression, and ongoing maintenance. Specific information on clinical trials is included with the relevant sections of chapters 8–10.

Table 7-2. Bipolar Disorder:
Summary of Efficacy Evidence from RCTs [8]

Drug	Mania Monotherapy	Mania Combination Therapy	Depression	Mainte-nance
Lithium	++	++*	+*	++
Divalproex	++	++*	+/−*	+*
Carbamazepine	++*	ND*	+/−*	+/−*
Lamotrigine	−*	ND*	+*	++
Clozapine	ND*	ND*	ND*	+*
Olanzapine	++	+	++*	++
Risperidone	++	+	+/−*	ND*
Quetiapine	++	++	†*	ND*
Ziprasidone	++	+*	ND*	ND*
Aripiprazole	++	ND*	ND*	+*

++ = Two adequately powered trials with positive findings
+ = One adequately powered trial with positive findings
† = One adequately powered trial
+/− = One adequately powered trial with equivocal findings
− = One adequately powered trial with negative findings
ND = No data

*not FDA approved for this condition

Factors Influencing Medication Strategies

Factors affecting medication strategies include:

- Medication side effects

- Reproductive issues (pregnancy, post-partum, lactation)

- Comorbid medical conditions (e.g., heart, renal, or hepatic disease)

- Comorbid and associated psychiatric disorders

- Cultural and age-associated considerations

Medication Side Effects

Drugs used to treat bipolar disorder can have serious side effects. Detailed information on side effects common to antimanic agents appears in chapter 8, while chapter 9 presents similar information for medications used to treat bipolar depression.

Treatment strategies could vary based on side effect profiles depending on the specific patient's health and lifestyle realities. For example, when selecting an atypical antipsychotic, the physician would want to choose a medication with less weight gain side effects for lethargic and obese patients. In any case, patients need to understand the possible side effects and their significance before starting on any specific treatment.

Reproductive Issues

Throughout pregnancy as well as after delivery and during lactation, significant risks exist with antimanic pharmacological therapy, including risks associated with birth defects, medication discontinuation, and neonatal health.[7, 9-11] For example, lithium, valproate, and carbamazepine have teratogenic effects and should be avoided, if possible, during pregnancy and lactation.

In addition to the potential teratogenic effect of the mood stabilizers, there is also concern that interrupting therapy may precipitate a mood episode. Therefore, when the patient elects to become pregnant or has discovered that she is pregnant, the patient, father, and clinicians (primary care, obstetrician, psychiatrist) must work together to assess the risks/benefits of continuing medication versus options such as cessation of pharmacotherapy during the gestation period or interruption during the first trimester.

Comorbid Medical Conditions

The presence of a comorbid medical condition interacts with bipolar disorder and its treatment in at least four ways:

1. Medical conditions can exacerbate bipolar disorder.

2. Bipolar disorder can exacerbate a medical condition.

3. Treatments for medical conditions can exacerbate bipolar disorder.

4. Treatments for bipolar disorder can exacerbate medical conditions.

The presence of a general medical condition may affect the results of pharmacotherapy of patients with bipolar disorder. For example, diuretics, angiotensin-converting enzyme inhibitors, nonsteroidal anti-inflammatory drugs, and low-salt diets all alter the excretion of lithium.[7] Essential drugs that affect cardiac conduction and rhythm or alter the function of organ systems involved in drug excretion may all limit the choice of medication. HIV-infected patients with bipolar disorder are at increased risk of drug-related adverse events because of their altered immune status and the potential for drug-drug interactions created by the spectrum of drugs used to treat the infection and prevent complications.

Monitoring for potential drug interactions between medications for bipolar disorder and medical conditions is also an important issue in illness management. These potential drug interactions include over-the-counter medications. For example, drugs taken for heart, renal, endocrinologic, or hepatic disease may interact with a mood stabilizer like lithium or other antimanic or antidepressive medications.

In part because of medication side effects, patients with bipolar disorder are at greater risk for cardiovascular disease, cancer, obesity, and type 2 diabetes mellitus compared with the general population. Meanwhile, patients with bipolar disorder are just as susceptible to these and other common medical illnesses as the general population. The increased risk for obesity and type 2 diabetes, which can be exacerbated by weight gain from some bipolar disorder treatments, suggests that monitoring of body weight, calculation of body mass index (BMI), and education about sound diet, nutrition, and exercise are important components of treatment.[12]

In addition, baseline and at least annual screening for hyperglycemia and dyslipidemias are important, especially in the presence of other risk factors for diabetes and the metabolic syndrome (e.g., hypertension, family history of diabetes, age, ethnicity, physical inactivity). These are general recommendations regardless of the medication regimen of the patient.

At the 2004 Consensus Development Conference on Antipsychotic Drugs and Obesity and Diabetes, experts from the American Diabetes Association, American Psychiatric Association, Association of Clinical Endocrinologists, and the North American Association for the Study of Obesity proposed a monitoring protocol for patients taking atypical antipsychotic medications. Table 7-3 below illustrates that protocol:[13]

Table 7-3. Monitoring Protocol for
Patients Taking Atypical Antipsychotics*[13]

Screening Measures	Baseline	4 Weeks	8 Weeks	12 Weeks	Quarterly	Annually	Every 5 Years
Personal/ family history	X					X	
Weight (BMI)	X	X	X	X	X		
Waist circumference	X			X		X	
Blood pressure	X			X		X	
Fasting plasma glucose	X			X		X	
Fasting lipid profile	X			X			X

* More frequent assessments may be warranted based on clinical status.
  (from American Diabetes Association et. al., 2004)

Comorbid and Associated Psychiatric Disorders

For patients with bipolar disorder and comorbid psychiatric symptoms, the current approach recommended in all APA and national guidelines is to treat comorbid symptoms with recommended treatments following remission of bipolar symptoms.

Substance Abuse

Comorbid substance abuse can significantly complicate therapy for patients with bipolar disorder. For example, inhibition of antidiuretic hormone by alcohol can predispose patients to dehydration and the potential for lithium toxicity. Chronic liver disease in patients with alcoholism or chronic hepatitis C can alter the pharmacokinetics of valproate and carbamazepine.

> *The course of illness for bipolar disorder with comorbid substance abuse is often more severe.*

Though there are few studies, some evidence suggests that anticonvulsant mood stabilizers, such as divalproex and carbamazepine, may be better than lithium for this population and may also improve treatment compliance.[14,15] Other studies suggest that increased patient contact, at the rate of up to two clinical contacts per week, as well as psychosocial support (group meetings and counseling) may also help improve patient outcomes and decrease hospitalizations and positive drug screens.[16]

Comorbid Anxiety Disorder

The treatment of comorbid anxiety disorder in bipolar disorder presents a challenge to clinicians. The most common method of treating anxiety disorders, usually tricyclics (TCA) or selective serotonin reuptake inhibitors (SSRIs), can result in the development of mania or hypomania in bipolar patients.[17] Clinicians should first stabilize the bipolar disorder with mood stabilizers before cautiously beginning a treatment regimen for the anxiety disorder with anxiolytics.[18]

Although lithium is commonly prescribed for bipolar disorder, a review of research suggests that valproate may sometimes be a good choice for comorbid anxiety, as it appears to improve symptoms in patients with panic disorder and OCD.[19] A recent review of atypical antipsychotic studies shows that these drugs, in addition to their mood stabilizing properties, also may have anxiolytic effects in patients with anxiety disorders, including OCD, PTSD, and GAD.[20] However, few studies currently exist that directly examine the treatment of comorbid anxiety and bipolar disorders. Studies completed suggest patients with comorbid anxiety disorders may respond less well to long-term treatment and suffer greater functional impairment.[21]

Associated Psychotic Symptoms

Psychotic manifestations may occur during a manic episode. If mild, antipsychotic drugs may not be required, and lithium or another agent may be adequate. If severe, an atypical antipsychotic can be administered during the acute phase and continued during maintenance therapy. Approximately one third of patients with bipolar mania may show catatonic symptoms, such as motor excitement, mutism, and stereotypic movements. Although ECT appears to be the most effective intervention in patients with catatonic features, lorazepam may also be effective and can be prescribed before other options.[22, 23]

Cultural and Age-Associated Concerns

Variations in drug metabolism related to race and ethnicity are cultural considerations that may affect drug dosage levels and responses. For example, Chinese patients have lower average activities of CYP2D6 and 2C9 than Caucasians.

Pharmacotherapy for elderly patients with bipolar disorder requires special care because these patients have reduced dose requirements, alterations in drug pharmacokinetics associated with renal or hepatic disease, and higher risks for drug-induced cognitive impairment, extrapyramidal side effects, such as tardive dyskinesia, orthostatic hypotension, and falls.[7]

Age-associated changes in renal clearance and volume of distribution generally reduce the dose requirements for lithium and other psychoactive drugs in the elderly.[7, 24] Associated chronic renal or hepatic disease can also alter the pharmacokinetics of drugs used to treat patients with bipolar illness. However, in the absence of side effects or demonstrable efficacy in an elderly patient, the dose of the drug should be slowly increased until it is in the therapeutic range. Elderly patients with bipolar disorder are also at a higher risk than younger patients for drug-induced cognitive impairment and extrapyramidal side effects.

Elderly patients may have increased end-organ sensitivity that increases both their response and the risk of side effects.

Psychosocial Therapy

Psychosocial interventions are appropriate measures to help the patient deal with disease-related issues, self-esteem, and adherence to treatment. Although focused psychosocial therapy may be effective in patients with acute bipolar depression, it fails to reduce manic symptoms, even when combined with pharmacotherapy.

Chapter 11 details efficacy studies on the use of psychosocial treatments.

Psychosocial treatments are particularly indicated when:

- Patients need help understanding and accepting the need for long-term pharmacotherapy.

- It is an adjunct to pharmacotherapy as a stable component of the patient's overall therapeutic regimen.

- Patients refuse medications.

- Patients want to avoid antidepressant-related adverse events (e.g., agitation or rapid cycling).

- The patient is being treated in the maintenance phase of bipolar illness.

Electroconvulsive Therapy (ECT)

The use of ECT as maintenance therapy is appropriate for patients who have:[7]

- Been diagnosed as having refractory or severe acute bipolar mania or depression, particularly if psychotic features or suicidal ideation are also present

- Achieved remission to a major mood episode through ECT in the past

Controlled studies have demonstrated that ECT is superior to placebo and at least as effective as TCAs or MAOI therapy.[25] ECT has been shown to produce superior outcomes to combination therapy with lithium and haloperidol.[25] In addition, patients treated with ECT followed by lithium maintenance therapy improved more significantly than did patients treated during acute mania and in the maintenance phase with lithium alone.[26]

References

1. Suppes T, Dennehy EB. Evidence-based long-term treatment of bipolar II disorder, *J Clin Psychiatry*. 2002. 63 Suppl 10:29-33.

2. American Psychiatric Association, American Psychiatric Association Task Force on DSM-IV. *Diagnostic and statistical manual of mental disorders: DSM-IV-TR*. Washington, DC, American Psychiatric Association, 2000.

3. Suppes T, Dennehy EB, Swann AC, Bowden CL, Calabrese JR, Hirschfeld RM, Keck PE, Jr., Sachs GS, Crismon ML, Toprac MG, Shon SP. Report of the Texas Consensus Conference Panel on medication treatment of bipolar disorder 2000. *J Clin Psychiatry*. 2002; 63(4):288-99.

4. Sobo S. Mood stabilizers and mood swings: In search of a definition. *Psychiatric Times*. 1999; 26(10).

5. Sachs GS. Bipolar mood disorder: practical strategies for acute and maintenance phase treatment. *J Clin Psychopharmacol*. 1996; 16(2 Suppl 1):32S-47S.

6. Sachs GS, Printz DJ, Kahn DA, Carpenter D, Docherty JP. The Expert Consensus Guideline Series: Medication Treatment of Bipolar Disorder 2000. *Postgrad Med*. 2000; Spec No:1-104.

7. American Psychiatric Association: Practice guideline for the treatment of patients with bipolar disorder (revision). *Am J Psychiatry*. 2002; 159(4 Suppl):1-50.

8. Keck PE, JR., McElroy SL. Treatment of bipolar disorder. *Textbook of Psychopharmacology*. 3rd Edition. Nemeroff CB, Schatzberg AF, eds. American Psychiatric Publishing, Inc., Washington, DC, 2004.

9. Viguera AC, Nonacs R, Cohen LS, Tondo L, Murray A, Baldessarini RJ. Risk of recurrence of bipolar disorder in pregnant and nonpregnant women after discontinuing lithium maintenance. *Am J Psychiatry*. 2000; 157(2):179-84.

10. Use of psychoactive medication during pregnancy and possible effects on the fetus and newborn. Committee on Drugs. *American Academy of Pediatrics*. *Pediatrics*. 2000; 105(4 Pt 1):880-7.

11. Yonkers KA. Wisner KL. Stowe Z. Leibenluft E. Cohen L. Miller L. Manber R. Viguera A. Suppes T. Altshuler L. Perspectives - reviews and overviews - Management of bipolar disorder during pregnancy and the postpartum period 2004. *Am J of Psychiatry*. 161(4):608-20.

12. Citrome L, Jaffe A, Levine J, Allingham B, Robinson J. Relationship between antipsychotic medication treatment and new cases of diabetes among psychiatric inpatients. *Psychiatr Serv*. 2004 Sep; 55(9):1006-13.

13. American Diabetes Association, American Psychiatric Association, Association of Clinical Endocrinologists, and the North American Association for the Study of Obesity, Consensus Development Conference on Antipsychotic Drugs and Obesity and Diabetes. *Diabetes Care*. 2004 27:596-601

14. Goldberg JF. Garno JL. Leon AC. Kocsis JH. Portera L. A history of substance abuse complicates remission from acute mania in bipolar disorder. *J Clin Psychiatry*. 1999; 60(11):733-40.

15. Weiss RD, Greenfield SF, Najavits LM. Soto JA. Wyner D. Tohen M. Griffin ML. Medication compliance among patients with bipolar disorder and substance use disorders. *J Clin Psychiatry*. 1998; 59:172-174.

16. Sloan KL. Rowe G. Substance abuse and psychiatric illness: treatment experience. *Am J Drug Alcohol Abuse*. 1998; 24:589-601.

17. Perugi G, Toni C, Frare F, Travierso MC, Hantouche E, Akiskal HS. Obsessive-compulsive-bipolar comorbidity: a systematic exploration of clinical features and treatment outcome. *J Clin Psychiatry*. 2002; 63:1129-1134.

18. Sasson Y, Chopra M, Harrari E, Amitai K, Zohar J. Bipolar comorbidity: from diagnostic dilemmas to therapeutic challenge. *Int J Neuropsychopharmacol*. 2003; 6(2):139-44.

19. Freeman MP, Freeman SA, McElroy SL. The comorbidity of bipolar and anxiety disorders: prevalence, psychobiology, and treatment issues. *J Affective Disorders*. 2002; 68:1-23.

20. McIntyre R, Katzman M. The role of atypical antipsychotics in bipolar depression and anxiety disorders. *Bipolar Disord*. 2003; 5 Suppl 2:20-35.

21. Henry C, Van den Bulke D, Bellivier F, Etain B, Rouillon F, Leboyer M: Anxiety disorders in 318 bipolar patients: prevalence and impact on illness severity and response to mood stabilizer. *J Clin Psychiatry*. 2003; 64(3):331-5.

22. Hawkins JM, Archer KJ, Strakowski SM, Keck PE: Somatic treatment of catatonia. *Int J Psychiatry Med*. 1995; 25(4):345-69.

23. Bush G, Fink M, Petrides G, Dowling F, Francis A: Catatonia. II. Treatment with lorazepam and electroconvulsive therapy. *Acta Psychiatr Scand*. 1996; 93(2):137-43.

24. Sproule BA, Hardy BG, Shulman KI: Differential pharmacokinetics of lithium in elderly patients. *Drugs Aging*. 2000; 16(3):165-77.

25. Mukherjee S, Sackeim HA, Schnur DB: Electroconvulsive therapy of acute manic episodes: a review of 50 years' experience. *Am J Psychiatry*. 1994; 151(2):169-76.

26. Small JG, Klapper MH, Kellams JJ, Miller MJ, Milstein V, Sharpley PH, Small IF: Electroconvulsive treatment compared with lithium in the management of manic states. *Arch Gen Psychiatry*. 1988; 45(8):727-325.

Chapter 8: Antimanic Agents

Antimanic agents are used in the treatment of patients with bipolar disorder with either manic or mixed episodes. The primary goals of therapy with these agents (see table 8-1 on the next page) are to rapidly ameliorate symptoms, such as agitation, impulsivity, and aggression, so that the patient can return to a normal level of functioning. This chapter discusses medications found to be effective in the treatment of acute mania in patients with bipolar I disorder, with a summary chart followed by detailed narrative.

Four types of medications are used for antimanic therapy. Lithium has been the mainstay of treatment for acute mania since 1970, but some antiepileptic drugs (AEDs) and typical antipsychotics as well as atypical antipsychotic agents (sometimes called newer or second generation psychotropics) provide antimanic efficacy for patients

Chapter 8 at a Glance

Table 8-1. Antimanic Medications*

▲ **Lithium***
▲ **Divalproex sodium***
▲ **Carbamazepine**
▲ **Typical Antipsychotics**
  ◆ Chlorpromazine*
  ◆ Haloperidol
  ◆ Perphenazine
  ◆ Thioridazine
▲ **Atypical Antipsychotics**
  ◆ Olanzapine*
  ◆ Clozapine
  ◆ Risperidone*
  ◆ Quetiapine*
  ◆ Ziprasidone*
  ◆ Aripiprazole*

*These agents have been specifically approved by the **U.S. Food and Drug Administration** for the treatment of **acute bipolar mania**.

Among anticonvulsants, divalproex/valproate/valproic acid and carbamazepine have been studied the most extensively for their use in antimanic therapy. Typical antipsychotics (e.g., chlorpromazine) have antimanic efficacy, particularly in patients with significant agitation; however, because of their neurological and neuroendocrinological side effects, they have been largely supplanted by the atypical antipsychotics. Atypical antipsychotics share many pharmacodynamic and pharmacokinetic properties, although they all have different adverse effects. Six agents in this class are commercially available at present: clozapine, olanzapine, quetiapine, risperidone, ziprasidone, and aripiprazole.

Table 8-2 (on pages 8-4 through 8-5) summarizes information about dosing and administration for the most commonly prescribed antimanic agents. These include lithium, anticonvulsants, and six atypical antipsychotics (newer generation psychotropics).

Lithium

Lithium (Li^+) is a monovalent cation that shares some of the properties of other cations such as sodium (N^+) and potassium (K^+). Although trace amounts are present in animal tissues, the cation has no known physiological role. Lithium was first introduced for the treatment of mania in 1949; however, concerns about the known potential effects of lithium toxicity restrained American psychiatrists from using it until 1970.[1] Since that time, it has become a mainstay of treatment for patients with acute mania.

Clinical Trial Results

Lithium has been shown to be superior to placebo for the treatment of acute mania.[2] Lithium appears to be most effective in patients with elated or classical manic symptoms who lack a history of frequent mood episodes. It also appears to be less effective in patients with mixed (dysphoric) episodes, or rapid cycling.[3]

Pharmacology

Mechanism of Action

Although a number of cellular effects of lithium have been established, the precise mechanism behind the drug's mood stabilizing properties is unknown. Possible candidates include its effect upon protein kinases, G proteins, and/or inhibition of inositol monophosphatase.

Table 8-2. Antimanic Agent Administration

	Antimanic Agent	Dose Range *	Admin. Schedule
	Lithium	0.6/1.0–1.2 mEq/L	BID or QHS
Anticonvulsants	**Divalproex, valproate, valproic acid**	80–125 µg/mL (acute) 50–125 µg/mL (overall)	BID or QHS
	Carbamazepine (also available in a long-acting formula)	400–1600 (4–12 µg/mL)	BID
	Oxcarbazepine	600–2400	BID or TID
Newer Generation Psychotropics (Atypical Antipsychotics)	**Clozapine**	75–900	QHS
	Olanzapine	10–20	QHS
	Quetiapine	500–800	BID or QHS
	Risperidone	2–6	BID or QHS
	Ziprasidone	120–160	BID
	Aripiprazole	10–30	QHS

*Mg/d unless otherwise noted; maintenance doses may be lower.
**Side effects may be less with long-acting forms of medications.

Side Effects** and Other Concerns

Tremor, drowsiness, nausea/vomiting, increased urine output, muscle weakness, thirst, dry mouth, cognitive impairment. **Concerns:** (1) Risk of toxicity increases at lithium levels above 1.5 mEq/L. Above 2.0 mEq/L, life-threatening side effects may occur.

Nausea/vomiting, increased appetite with weight gain, sedation, hair loss, reversible increases in liver function tests, reversible thrombocytopenia, rarely pancreatitis and liver failure: **Concerns:** (1) Divalproex sodium, the enteric-coated form of valproate, is the FDA-approved form for treatment of acute mania.(2) Valproate can increase free warfarin levels and increase bleeding time. (3) Use of both drugs should be monitored carefully. Aspirin inhibits valproate metabolism.

Dizziness, drowsiness, double vision, fatigue, nausea, vomiting, ataxia, tremor, discomfort due to indigestion, abnormal gait, hyponatremia, rash; rare Stevens-Johnson Syndrome; agranulocytosis

Dizziness, hyponatremia, ataxia, diplopia, headache, sedation, impaired speech, double vision, nausea and gastrointestinal upset, reversible mild, below-normal white blood cell range. May lower oral contraceptive efficacy.

Sedation, weight gain***, dry mouth, constipation, and potential mental confusion, abrupt drop in blood pressure when suddenly changing from lying to sitting or sitting to standing, rapid heart rate, excessive salivation, constipation, nausea, and vomiting. **Concerns:** (1) Associated incidence of agranulocytosis; lowering of seizure threshold; May lower oral contraceptive efficacy.

Sedation, weight gain***, dry mouth, constipation, potential mental confusion, mild Parkinson-like symptoms (e.g., flat facial expression, stiff muscles, slowed movements)

Sedation, weight gain***, orthostatic hypotension

Sedation, Parkinson-like symptoms (e.g., flat facial expression, stiff muscles, slowed movements), weight gain,*** hypotension, prolactin elevation

Sedation, QTc prolongation, nausea, vomiting, constipation, Parkinson-like symptoms (e.g., flat facial expression, stiff muscles, slowed movements), dizziness. **Concerns:** (1) Should be taken with food.

Sedation, Parkinson-like symptoms (e.g., flat facial expression, stiff muscles, slowed movements), internal feeling of restlessness or agitation (akathisia)

***Severity of weight gain generally rated:
clozapine = olanzapine > quetiapine = risperidone > aripiprazole = ziprasidone.

Absorption, Metabolism, Excretion

Lithium is readily absorbed from the gastrointestinal tract; almost all administered drug enters the plasma within eight hours. Following an oral dose, peak plasma levels appear within two to four hours.[1] Since it is a small hydrophilic molecule, lithium's volume of distribution is approximately that of total body water. However, this volume is significantly less than that of other psychotropic drugs that are both lipophilic and protein bound. Lithium slowly passes through the blood-brain barrier, with final concentrations within the cerebrospinal fluid of 40 to 50 percent.

The drug is almost completely excreted by the kidneys; approximately one- to two-thirds is excreted within 12 hours of administration. Following glomerular filtration, approximately 80 percent of lithium is reabsorbed by the proximal convoluted tubules (PCT). Since it shares reabsorption with sodium, renal mechanisms will increase PCT lithium absorption in patients with decreased concentrations of sodium in the glomerular filtrate. Since plasma lithium is a function of the dose administered and the patient's renal function, plasma levels of the drug will remain remarkably constant in a given individual.

Side Effects

Table 8-3, on the next two pages, provides detailed information on management of common lithium side effects.

Table 8-3. Management of Side Effects Associated with Lithium

Side Effects/ Comments	Treatment Considerations
Postabsorptive syndrome — GI discomfort, nausea, weakness, vertigo • Due to a rapid rise in plasma lithium levels • Subsides over time	• Give all at bedtime. • Try alternative preparations.
Fine tremors of the hands, fatigue can be common and persistent	• Check serum level. • Use propranolol or similar medication.
Thirst, polydipsia, polyuria, low urine specific gravity • Drug-induced abnormalities in renal function caused by decreased renal response to antidiuretic hormone • Some patients may continue to have impaired concentrating ability • Nephrogenic diabetes insipidus may occur	• Polyuria can sometimes be managed by administering the drug once daily at bedtime. • Dose reduction may be needed to control symptoms. • Adequate fluid and electrolyte replacement may be needed. • Thiazide may be required for severe symptoms, but electrolytes should be monitored, potassium supplementation may be needed, and lithium dose should be reduced. • Potassium-sparing diuretics (e.g., amiloride) can be effective and will usually not increase potassium excretion or lithium reabsorption.
Interstitial fibrosis, glomerular sclerosis, impaired water reabsorption, increased serum creatinine • Associated with long-term lithium use in some instances	• Monitor kidney function initially and then biannually.

Table 8-3. (continued)

Side Effects/ Comments	Treatment Considerations
Repolarization abnormalities on electrocardiogram (ECG) —conduction block or arrhythmia in some instances	• ECG usually indicated prior to initiating in an individual over age 40.
Hypothyroidism • More common in women • Affects up to one third of patients treated with lithium • May appear after the patient has been treated for 6 to 18 months • May be accompanied by rapid cycling • Associated risk of depression for patients who develop lithium-induced hypothyroidism	• Levothyroxine can be used while patient is maintained on lithium. • Thyroid hormone replacement therapy and substitution of another mood stabilizer can be considered if rapid cycling or depression occur. • Thyroid stimulating hormone level should be checked one to two times per year.
Dermatologic changes—pustular acne, exacerbation or precipitation of psoriasis, inhibition of anti-psoriatic therapy[4]	• Treat empirically.

Drug Interactions

Many drugs can alter serum lithium levels:

- During the initial phases of therapy
- When the patient has a medical illness
- When the patient is treated with any type of new drug that can alter lithium excretion

In patients treated with lithium and an antipsychotic, the antiemetic activity of the drug can mask some of the gastrointestinal symptoms of lithium toxicity. Therefore, it is imperative that patients have their serum lithium levels monitored regularly. Such monitoring is particularly important. (See table 8-4 and the *Physicians Desk Reference* for a comprehensive list of drugs affecting serum lithium levels.)

Table 8-4. Drugs that Affect Serum Lithium Levels

Drug	Effect
Thiazides	⬆
Furosemide	⬆
Spironolactone	⬆
Methyldopa	⬆
Indomethacin	⬆
Phenylbutazone	⬆
Piroxicam	⬆
Ibuprofen	⬆
Acetazolamide	⬇
Sodium Bicarbonate	⬇
Sodium Chloride	⬇
Theophylline	⬇
Mannitol	⬇

Administration

Primary Considerations

Before treatment begins, the patient's history and physical examination should be reviewed to address any issues in organ systems likely to be affected by the drug (e.g., endocrine, cardiovascular, genitourinary, skin). The patient should also be educated about lithium's potential toxicities. For obvious reasons, laboratory studies should include baseline electrolytes, chemistry, urinalysis, renal function, pregnancy, thyroid-stimulating hormone, and electrocardiogram (when appropriate).

Dosage Selection

Selection of the total daily dose should be based upon age, weight, and other medical considerations. To minimize side effects, the total lithium dose is usually administered in three divided doses or at bedtime (QHS). The dose is usually kept low (e.g., 300-600 mg/d) and then titrated upward to the therapeutic target of 0.5 to 1.2 mmol/L. This usually requires 900 to 1800 mg/d (15 to 20 mg/kg).

In an attempt to balance side effects with therapeutic activity, lithium levels in the mid to upper range (0.8 to 1.2 mmol/L) are often required for the treatment of acute mania.

Titration

The rate of titration appears to affect the rapidity of response to lithium and other mood stabilizers.[2] While randomized clinical trials document symptomatic improvement within 7 to 14 days, a pilot study demonstrated that patients whose dose levels were rapidly titrated to therapeutic concentrations within 24 hours experienced a significant reduction in symptoms within a span of five days.[5]

Long-Term Management

During the first six months of therapy, lithium levels should be monitored regularly, and renal and thyroid function also should be assessed. In a stable and responsible patient, testing can then be reduced to biannually unless breakthrough occurs, toxic manifestations develop, a general medical condition intervenes, or the patient's medication changes.

Toxicity

Lithium toxicity is related to serum drug levels and is most common with serum lithium levels of 1.5 mmol/L or greater.[6] Potentially life-threatening side effects are common when drug levels exceed 2.0 mmol/L. At lower levels, manifestations of toxicity are those described under adverse events. At higher concentrations, however, symptoms increase in severity and may be accompanied by neurologic impairments, seizures, coma, and cardiac arrhythmias. The risk of adverse effects is not only a function of the serum lithium levels; it is also affected by the duration of exposure to the high levels.

Anticonvulsants

Anticonvulsants found to have mood stabilizing properties include: valproate, carbamazepine, and lamotrigine (in maintenance use).

Potential mechanisms of action of anticonvulsants in bipolar disorder include.

- Altering sodium and potassium fluxes via ion channels
- Upregulation of inhibitory and downregulation of excitatory neurotransmitters
- Downregulation of excitatory neurotransmitters
- Modulation of second messenger systems

Divalproex/Valproate/Valproic Acid

Valproic acid is a simple, branched-chain carboxylic acid. Its anticonvulsant properties were discovered when it was used as a vehicle for drugs being screened for antiepileptic activity.

Clinical Trial Results

Divalproex sodium is indicated for the treatment of the manic episodes associated with bipolar disorder. Valproic acid and related formulations have superior efficacy compared with placebo and comparable activity with lithium, haloperidol, and olanzapine.[2] Factors associated with improved valproate versus lithium response include mixed episodes and a history of multiple prior mood episodes. The effect of valproate in comparison trials of antipsychotic compounds suggests that, like all antimanic agents, valproate has antipsychotic as well as antimanic activity.

Pharmacology

The basis for valproate's mood stabilizing properties is not fully understood. However, since it blocks ion channels, it is thought that valproate may possibly upregulate the activity of GABAergic and downregulate the activity of glutamatergic neurotransmitters.[1]

Absorption, Metabolism, Excretion — Following oral administration, valproate is rapidly absorbed, and peak serum levels are achieved within one to four hours. Once it enters the bloodstream, the drug is rapidly distributed throughout the body and extensively protein bound. Its half-life is typically in the six- to 16-hour range, but it can be significantly altered by drugs that interfere with the activities of hepatic cytochromes, such as CYP2C9, or the process of conjugation of the drug to glucuronic acid. Once conjugated with glucuronic acid, valproate and its metabolites are predominantly excreted through the urine. Since one valproate metabolite is eliminated in the urine, its presence may register as a ketone and lead to a false positive of urinary ketones.

Side Effects

Table 8-5, on the next page, summarizes valproate side effect management.

Table 8-5. Management of Side Effects
Associated with Valproate

Side Effects/Comments	Treatment Considerations
Sedation and GI distress common at start of treatment; symptoms usually resolve over time	• Manage persistent, drug-associated GI distress by dose reduction, switch to another member of the valproate family (e.g., divalproex sodium for sodium valproate), and/or administer an H_2-receptor blocker (e.g., cimetidine).
Hair loss, weight gain, increased appetite	• Recommend diet and exercise. • Consider agents associated with weight loss (e.g., topiramate, zonisamide).
Mild leucopenia, thrombocytopenia, impaired platelet function	• Conduct baseline complete blood count. • Determine platelet counts and bleeding time before elective surgery and if patient has excessive bruising or hemorrhage.
Tremors may occur	• Treat with a β-blocker (e.g., propranolol).
May increase incidence of polycystic ovarian syndrome Rate of development lower than initially reported[7, 8, 9]	• Treat with oral contraceptives.
Abnormal liver function, hyperammonemia in severe cases occurs in some patients	• Monitor liver function tests monthly at treatment outset, then biannually.
Hepatocellular necrosis, hemorrhagic pancreatitis, and agranulocytosis Rare idiosyncratic reactions	• Patients should be advised to seek medical help if they develop abdominal pain, jaundice, acute pharyngitis with fever, bleeding or purpura.

Drug Interactions: Aspirin, Warfarin, Lamotrigine — Valproate can interact with a number of medications. Since the drug is largely protein bound, it can displace other drugs from serum proteins (e.g., aspirin and warfarin). Since valproate can impair non-renal clearance of barbiturates, barbiturate drug levels should be obtained for patients receiving both drugs, and they should be monitored for signs of neurological toxicity. Valproate inhibits the metabolism of lamotrigine; consequently, the lamotrigine dose in patients concurrently treated with valproate must be started at a dose one half that of the recommended initial dose.

Administration

Preliminary considerations — Before treatment begins, the patient should undergo a comprehensive medical examination to detect evidence of preexisting hepatic or hematologic abnormalities. Baseline liver function tests and complete blood count should also be obtained.

Dosage selection — Valproate has a comparatively wide therapeutic index compared with lithium.[2] Acute antimanic activity is in the range of 50 to 125 mg/L, with improved response rates at the upper end of the therapeutic range. While some patients may require drug levels in excess of 125 mg/L to control their symptoms, side effects progressively increase above this level. Data from clinical trials indicate that divalproex therapy can be initiated safely at a dose of 20 to 30 mg/kg/d in hospitalized patients.[6] To minimize gastrointestinal and neurological toxicities, valproate treatment of outpatients is usually started at a dose of 250 mg three times a day or QHS (total dose = 750 mg/d).

Titration — Depending on the clinical response and side effects, the initial dose can be titrated upward every few days until drug levels are in the therapeutic range. However, the maximal daily adult dose should not exceed 60 mg/kg/d. Since many patients do well with once- or twice-daily dosing, the treatment regimen can be simplified when the patient is stabilized.

An extended release formulation of divalproex is now available that allows for once-daily dosing and apparently reduces the incidence of side effects. However, since the bioavailability of the extended release formulation is only approximately 85 percent of the immediate-release formulation, some patients must be treated with slightly higher doses.

Carbamazepine

Carbamazepine is chemically related to the tricyclic antidepressants. Although initially approved for the treatment of seizures, it has also been used to treat patients with various pain syndromes, such as trigeminal neuralgia. Although the drug has been used in combination with lithium for many years in Europe for the treatment of acute mania, large, placebo-controlled, randomized clinical trials have only recently been completed with the extended-release formulation.[8] Carbamazepine has been shown to have antimanic activity in some patients who are refractory to lithium.

Clinical Trial Results

Although superior to placebo in the treatment of acute mania, carbamazepine is often considered a second-line antimanic agent, principally because, until recently, there are few well designed, randomized controlled trials of its use in mania.[2] Several trials have shown its efficacy to be comparable to that of lithium. However, a recent small comparative study found that the drug has less antimanic efficacy than valproate.[9] Because of the superior pharmacokinetics and tolerability of oxcarbazepine, it is often substituted for carbamazepine.

Pharmacology

Carbamazepine's antiepileptic activity is similar to phenytoin.[1] Once administered, it inhibits repolarization by downregulating the recovery rate of voltage-activated sodium channels.

Absorption, Metabolism, Excretion — Carbamazepine is slowly absorbed from the gastrointestinal tract, with peak levels four to 24 hours after a single dose. Once it enters the plasma, the majority of the drug is bound to serum proteins; approximately 20 to 30 percent of carbamazepine circulates in its free form and rapidly equilibrates in tissues. The drug is metabolized in the liver, conjugated with glucuronic acid, and excreted into the urine. Its elimination half-life is approximately 36 hours. With regular administration, however, carbamazepine upregulates the activity of hepatic enzymes, with a resultant decrease in the half-life to 16 to 24 hours.

Oxcarbazepine is a prodrug. It is a less potent inducer of hepatic enzymes; consequently, it increases plasma levels of valproate. Additionally, unlike carbamazepine where the metabolite is responsible for toxicity and side effects, oxcarbazepine metabolites are generally nontoxic. However, while similar, it is pharmacologically a different drug and direct tests of its efficacy in bipolar disorder are needed.

Side Effects

Table 8-6, on the following page, provides detailed information on common carbamazepine side effects.

Drug Interactions — Drugs that increase activity of hepatic cytochromes CYP3A4, such as valproate, increase the metabolism and lower serum carbamazepine levels.[1] Like its tricyclic relatives, carbamazepine has anticholinergic activity that can lead to adverse events — dryness of the mouth, constipation, diplopia, blurred vision, etc.

Carbamazepine reduces plasma concentrations and efficacy of the typical antipsychotic, haloperidol. Fluoxetine, some antibiotics, and calcium channel blockers inhibit carbamazepine metabolism.

Administration

Preliminary Considerations — Before treatment begins, patients require a thorough medical history and examination to rule out preexisting disorders, including liver and blood diseases. Laboratory studies should include liver function tests, a complete blood count, and electrolytes.

**Table 8-6. Side Effects
Associated with Carbamazepine**

Side Effects	Comments
CNS—drowsiness, headache	Most common
GI tract—nausea and vomiting	Dose and/or level to be checked; once daily dosing considered
Dermatological	Non-medically serious rash; potentially fatal Stevens-Johnson syndrome and toxic epidermal necrolysis reported (rare)
Hematologic, hepatic, cardiovascular, and cutaneous reactions	Most serious
Leukopenia	Mild, transient leukopenia in approximately 10% of patients; persistent leukopenia in approximately 2%, requiring drug discontinuation[1]
Fatal aplastic anemia	Approximately 1/200,000 patients
Transient elevation of hepatic enzymes	Approximately 5–10% of patients
Cardiac conduction abnormalities— bradycardia, arrhythmias, or complete heart block	Baseline ECG in patients age 45 or older

Dosage Selection — There is an inconstant relationship between the dose of carbamazepine, serum concentration, response, and side effects. Therefore, in adults, treatment is usually started at a total daily dose of 200–600 mg, divided into three or four doses.[6] While the dose can be increased in hospitalized patients in increments of 200 mg/d up to 800–1000 mg/d, slower dosage adjustments are usually indicated for less severly ill outpatients. Target serum concentrations for those with bipolar disorder have not been established; therefore, most clinicians try to maintain serum carbamazepine levels

Signs of Carbamazepine Toxicity:

- *Dizziness*
- *Ataxia*
- *Nystagmus*
- *Extrapyramidal signs*
- *Sedation*
- *Stupor*
- *Respiratory difficulties*
- *Arrhythmias*
- *Cardiac conduction abnormalities*
- *Coma*
- *Convulsions*

in the 4–12 µg/mL range. Since side effects are primarily due to the metabolite of carbamazepine, in some patients this can occur at low serum levels and in others at much higher serum levels. During the first two months of therapy, hematologic parameters and liver function tests should be monitored frequently.

Other Anticonvulsants

A number of other anticonvulsants have been studied as potential antimanic agents. These include gabapentin, lamotrigine, topiramate, zonisamide, levetiracetam, tiagabine, and acamprosate. Studies of these drugs have been limited by sample size and methodologic issues. However, placebo-controlled studies with lamotrigine and topiramate in acute bipolar mania were negative.[2]

Typical Antipsychotics

Typical antipsychotics include haloperidol, chlorpromazine, thioridazine, and perphenazine. These medications have antimanic efficacy, particularly in patients with significant agitation.[10] However, their side effects limit their long-term use. These include increased risk of depression, prolactin elevation, and extrapyramidal manifestations, such as tardive dyskinesia in patients with bipolar disorder. Therefore, they have been largely supplanted by the atypical antipsychotics.

Atypical Antipsychotics
(Newer Generation Psychotropics)

Atypical antipsychotic agents are the newest additions to the psychotropic class and are remarkable for their overall improved side-effect profile. However, patients treated with antipsychotics are still at risk for extrapyramidal side effects: akathisia, tardive dyskinesia, and neuroleptic malignant syndrome. The degree of this risk has not yet been fully defined and may vary across the agents in this class.

Characteristics of these newer generation psychotropics are:

1. Minimal-to-no extrapyramidal side effects

2. Intrinsic antimanic properties

3. Different receptor affinities
   a) D_1, D_3, D_4 >D_2;
   b) $5-HT_{2A}$ >D_2

4. Less potential for the neuroleptic malignant syndrome

5. Greater efficacy than typical agents in some types of schizophrenia (e.g., schizophrenic deficit symptoms)

6. Beneficial effects in the treatment of depressive symptoms (some atypicals)

Overall Side Effects

Atypical antipsychotics (newer generation psychotropics) have varying side effect profiles related to weight gain, glucose intolerance, hyperprolactinemia, QTc prolongation, somnolence, orthostatic hypotension, and extrapyramidal symptoms (see table 8-7 on the next page).

The side effects of atypical antipsychotics are less than with typical antipsychotics.

Table 8-7. Comparative Side Effect Profile of Atypical Antipsychotics[11-18]

Side Effects	Atypical Antipsychotics					
	Clozapine	Olanzapine	Risperidone	Quetiapine	Ziprasidone	Aripiprazole
Weight Gain*	3+	3+	2+	2+	+	+
Hyperprolactinemia	±	±	3+	±	±	–
Somnolence	3+	2+	+	2+	+	+
QTc Prolongation	2+	±	±	±	+	±
Orthostatic Hypotension	3+	+	2+	2+	2+	+
Extrapyramidal Symptoms	±	±	2+	±	+	+

3+ = high incidence
2+ = moderate incidence
1+ = low incidence
± = equivocal findings
– = insignificant incidence
*Also associated with dyslipidemia

General Treatment Recommendations

- Advise patients about the identification and significance of these side effects prior to administering medication.

- Obtain baseline glucose and lipid profiles when therapy is started and then monitor at least annually. (See page 7-21 for recommended monitoring schedule.)

- Treat the triad of weight gain, glucose intolerance, and dyslipidemia the same as for patients with the metabolic syndrome.

- Advise patients to lose weight and increase physical activity.

- Address other cardiovascular risk factors, such as increased LDL-C, low HDL-C, hypertension, and cigarette smoking.

- Analyze the risk-benefit of switching to another drug in a patient whose psychiatric disorder is well controlled.

Other clinical considerations and specific treatment recommendations for the common side effects of atypical antipsychotics are listed in Table 8-8. Management of Side Effects of Atypical Antipsychotics on pages 8-23 through 8-26.

Weight gain — This complication is the result of drug-induced alterations in neurotransmitter circuitry involved in feeding behavior and satiety. The strongest correlation is the affinity of the drug for H_1 and possibly 5-HT_{2C} receptors. The actions of the former may be due to a blockade of satiety signals from the gut, while the latter appears to act by stimulating food intake. Another possible mechanism is interference with the leptin-mediated feeding behavior and total body mass of adipose tissue.

> *Patients usually report an increase in appetite. Not all patients gain weight. The most effective strategies are diet and exercise.*

Glucose intolerance — This effect is probably multifactorial. Possible mechanisms include weight-gain associated insulin resistance, 5-HT_{1A}-antagonist-mediated hypoinsulinemia, and one or both of the aforementioned effects in those predisposed to the disease because of race or other genetic/environmental factors.

Dyslipidemia — Although the etiology of dyslipidemia is unknown, it is presumably related to weight gain and insulin resistance, factors also associated with the metabolic syndrome.

Hyperprolactinemia — The antidopaminergic activity of the atypical antipsychotics can remove the tonic dopamine-induced inhibition of prolactin secretion by the pituitary.

QTc Prolongation — The QTc segment of the ECG reflects the repolarization phase of the cardiac cycle. Atypical antipsychotics and a number of other drugs, as well as acquired and inherited disorders, can prolong repolarization; this effect is reflected in a prolonged QTc interval.[19] Prolongation of repolarization can be accompanied by spatial dispersion of repolarization. As a result, individual cardiac muscle fibers become responsive to electrical impulses at different times.

Neuroleptic malignant syndrome (NMS) — Manifestations of NMS are believed to be due to either blockade of dopaminergic receptors or withdrawal of exogenous dopaminergic agonists. Therefore, the probability is directly related to the antidopaminergic activity of the antipsychotic agent.

Table 8-8. Management of Side Effects
of Atypical Antipsychotics (AAPs)

Side Effect	Clinical Considerations	Treatment Recommendations
Weight gain	Most AAPs are associated with significant weight gain. Clozapine and olanzapine appear to induce the most weight gain. Some evidence suggests that the weight plateau differs among agents and that weight may stabilize within the first few months. Patients should be encouraged to follow healthy eating habits and exercise regularly. There does not appear to be a clear correlation between weight gain and drug dose or severity of disease.	• Patients should be weighed at each visit and questioned about an increase in clothes or belt size. • They should be given advice on dietary/physical activity as well.
DysLipidemia	Patients treated with AAPs can develop hypertriglyceridemia.[19]	• Since hypertriglyceridemia is an independent risk factor for coronary heart disease, lipid monitoring is an important element of care.
	Reported increases in serum triglycerides range from 10–50% or greater.	
	Most reports have described this association with clozapine or olanzapine, drugs also associated with the most significant weight gain and glucose intolerance. However, cases of dyslipidemia have been described with other members of this class.	

Side Effect	Clinical Considerations	Treatment Recommendations
Hyperprolactinemia	Antidopaminergic activity of AAPs can remove the tonic dopamine-induced inhibition of prolactin secretion by the pituitary. This effect appears to be most common with risperidone and may or may not be symptomatic.[19]	
	Clinical manifestations include galactorrhea, gynecomastia, amenorrhea, anovulation, impaired spermatogenesis, decreased libido, anorgasmia, and impotence.	• Patients should be asked about prolactin-related symptoms during follow-up examinations.
	Routine screening for this side effect is not indicated.	• Prolactin levels should be assayed in symptomatic patients and, if elevated, treated.
		• Dopaminergic agonists, such as bromocriptine, can be used to manage this condition, but they have the potential to worsen the psychiatric disorder. • The best approach is usually to switch to another AAP.

Side Effect	Clinical Considerations	Treatment Recommendations
QTc prolongation	AAPs (e.g., ziprasidone) and a number of other drugs, as well as acquired and inherited disorders, have the potential to prolong repolarization; this effect is reflected in a prolonged QTc interval.[19]	• Obtain a baseline ECG, electrolytes, and tests of renal and hepatic function when starting patients on ziprasidone if they are at risk for prolonged QTc.
	Consequences of the disordered cardiac electrophysiology include arrhythmias, such as ventricular tachycardia and torsades de pointes.	• Treatment consists of correcting electrolyte abnormalities, discontinuing non-essential medications that may also prolong the interval; lastly, another drug can be substituted for the offending agent.
	Risk of torsades de pointes increases when the QTc interval is greater than 500 ms.	
	Risk of arrhythmias is increased in patients with other metabolic derangements (e.g., hypokalemia or hypomagnesemia)	

Side Effect	Clinical Considerations	Treatment Recommendations
Neuroleptic malignant syndrome	An idiosyncratic reaction to antipsychotic agents. Risk factors may include agitation, dehydration, and IM administration (e.g., typical antipsychotics).	• Treatment consists of rapid cooling with fluid and electrolyte support.
	Manifested by hyperthermia, muscle rigidity, altered mental status, tremors, and manifestations of autonomic dysfunction (e.g., blood pressure lability, cardiac arrhythmias, and diaphoresis).	• If the patient does not respond to cooling measures, bromocriptine (a dopamine antagonist) or dantrolene (a calcium-blocking skeletal muscle relaxant) may be required.
	Usually occurs within several days of onset of therapy with drug levels within the therapeutic range.	• Antipyretics are not indicated.
	Untreated, the course may be complicated by myocardial infarction, respiratory failure, mixed respiratory and metabolic acidosis, rhabdomyolysis, and acute renal failure.	

Newer Generation Psychotropic Medications

Six atypical antipsychotics are now commercially available: clozapine, olanzapine, quetiapine, risperidone, ziprasidone, and aripiprazole. These atypical antipsychotics share many pharmacodynamic and pharmacokinetic properties.

Clozapine

Mechanism of Action — Clozapine has a complex receptor profile including dopaminergic and serotonergic as well as some muscarinic, histaminic, and adrenergic activity. The dual action of activity at dopaminergic and serotonergic receptors is what led to the explosion of development of the atypical antipsychotics. Prior to clozapine the older generation antipsychotics activity focused on dopamine receptors only. Clozapine's serotonergic activity led to a major reconceptualization in the field.

Clozapine was the first atypical antipsychotic. Although a useful agent, the side effect and associated incidence of agranulocytosis make it impractical as a first-line agent for most patients. This medication, however, is an important second-line agent for patients who have failed other atypical antipsychotics and are treatment resistant.

Clinical Trial Results — A randomized trial comparing clozapine with chlorpromazine in hospitalized patients with acute mania reported no significant differences in efficacy between the two drugs, although the trial was insufficiently powered to detect a difference at study endpoint.[20] However, results did suggest that clozapine may have a more rapid onset of action. In an uncontrolled trial for treatment-resistant mania, clozapine was efficacious.[21]

Dosage Selection — On the first day of treatment, one or two 25-mg tablets are usually administered with the initial oral dose not to exceed 75 mg. If well tolerated, the dosage may be increased daily in increments of 25–50 mg, so that a target dose of 300–450 mg/d is reached by the end of two weeks. In maintenance, long-term daily dosage ranges from 100–450 mg/d.[22]

Olanzapine

Mechanism of Action — Olanzapine has complex receptor activities with serotonergic, dopaminergic as well as muscarinic, histaminic, and alpha adrenergic activity.

Olanzapine is the most extensively studied of the atypical antipsychotics in patients with acute mania. It was the first atypical antipsychotic to receive US Food and Drug Administration (FDA) approval for this indication. When it was approved, it was redesignated as a psychotropic drug by the FDA as an attempt to describe its activity outside of psychotic disorders.

Clinical Trial Results — The efficacy of olanzapine for acute bipolar mania has been established in at least six randomized clinical trials.[23] Its efficacy has been established versus placebo, divalproex, and haloperidol. The drug was superior to placebo, at least as effective as divalproex, and comparable to haloperidol without associated worsening of depressive symptom scores during mania. The intramuscular preparation has been shown to be effective in the management of agitation in patients with acute bipolar mania.

Dosage Selection — When administered in combination with lithium or valproate, olanzapine therapy for acute bipolar mania should generally be started at 10 mg once a day. In studies of short-term therapy, antimanic efficacy was present in a dose range of 5–20 mg/d.

Quetiapine

Mechanism of Action — Quetiapine has receptor activity at serotonergic, dopaminergic and, to a lesser degree, at alpha adrenergic and histaminic receptors.

Clinical Trials Results — Four randomized, controlled trials have demonstrated that quetiapine exerts antimanic activity.[23] As monotherapy, it is superior to placebo for acute mania symptom control. Similarly, quetiapine in combination with lithium or divalproex was superior to placebo in reducing manic symptoms. Additionally patients sustained antimanic effects at week 12 of therapy. [24]

Dosage Selection — In the latter three clinical trials described above, quetiapine was given in increasing doses of 100mg/d for the first four days, followed by 600 mg/d on day five and 800 mg/d on day six. The average dose in responders was approximately 600 mg/d in divided doses in both the monotherapy and adjunct therapy trials**.**

Risperidone

Risperidone differs from the other atypical antipsychotics in that the drug has a relatively greater affinity at dopaminergic terminals than the other agents. This effect is manifested in a dose-dependant manner in a tuberoinfundibular dopaminergic pathway by associated hyperprolactinemia.

Clinical Trial Results — Placebo-controlled trials of risperidone and haloperidol combined with lithium, divalproex, or carbamazepine indicate that both drugs are superior to placebo and equally efficacious. In addition, in conventional doses, treatment with risperidone was accompanied by fewer extrapyramidal symptoms than with haloperidol.[23] Two, placebo-controlled monotherapy trials also demonstrated the efficacy of risperidone in acute bipolar mania.

Dosage selection — In patients with acute bipolar mania, risperidone can be administered once a day, starting with 2–3 mg/d. The dose can be then adjusted in increments of 1 mg/d. Antimanic activity is reported to be in the 1–6 mg/d range, with usual antimanic dose of 4–6 mg/d.

Ziprasidone

Ziprasidone has a mechanism similar to that of other atypical antipsychotics but produces more extensive blockade of the serotonergic receptors. It also appears to block the serotonin and norepinephrine transporters to some degree. Since ziprasidone may produce QTc prolongation, coadministration with other drugs or metabolic abnormalities that significantly prolong the QT interval have the potential to produce arrhythmias, including the potentially fatal torsades de pointes.

Clinical Trial Results — Studies of ziprasidone in patients with acute bipolar mania demonstrated that the drug is superior to placebo and equivalent in efficacy, but has fewer side effects than haloperidol.[23]

Dosage Selection — Oral ziprasidone should be started at an initial, twice-daily dose of 40 mg taken with food. The daily dosage may subsequently be adjusted at intervals of at least one day, up to 80 mg twice a day, on the basis of the patient's individual clinical status.

Aripiprazole

Aripiprazole is a newer atypical antipsychotic. Its mechanism of action is as a partial dopamine D_2 agonist.

Clinical Trial Results — In studies of patients with acute mania, aripiprazole had superior efficacy compared with placebo and was at least as effective as haloperidol, without the latter's associated extrapyramidal adverse effects.[23]

Dosage Selection — Aripiprazole is administered at a starting dose of 15–30 mg/d for patients with acute mania. Maintenance and outpatient dosage may be lower.

Topiramate and Lamotrigine

Chapter 9 includes a detailed review of lamotrigine (pages 9-4 through 9-5) and topiramate (pages 9-7 through 9-8).

Antimanic Combination Therapy

To date, most accumulated data about antimanic combination therapy come from studies of lithium, valproate, and olanzapine. At present, lithium and/or valproate have been studied in combination with haloperidol, olanzapine, risperidone, quetiapine, or ziprasidone.[2] Although trials have not addressed dosing issues of monotherapy versus combination therapy, no data suggest that the standard doses should be adjusted when mood stabilizers of different classes are given in combination.

Treatment with two mood stabilizing agents has been demonstrated to have a more rapid onset of action and greater efficacy than monotherapy in patients with acute bipolar mania.[2, 25, 26] Although there have been no randomized controlled trials, anecdotal reports suggest that the combination of lithium plus valproate is more efficacious than monotherapy with either agent.[27] Studies have demonstrated that combination therapy is particularly valuable in patients with severe symptoms or psychotic features.[6]

The efficacy of lithium appears to be less robust in patients with mixed episodes (mania with a minimum of depressive symptoms).[8] In contrast, studies support valproate, risperidone, ziprasidone, aripriprazole, and olanzapine as agents with comparable efficacy in both manic and mixed episodes.[3, 28] Of the other antimanic drugs, only carbamazepine has been reported to produce responses in patients with mixed episodes.[29]

References

1. Goodman LS, Hardman JG, Limbird LE, Gilman AG. *Goodman & Gilman's the pharmacological basis of therapeutics.* New York: McGraw-Hill; 2001.

2. Keck PE, JR., McElroy SL. Treatment of bipolar disorder. *Textbook of Psychopharmacology*, 3rd Edition. Nemeroff CB, Schatzberg AF, eds. American Psychiatric Publishing, Inc. Washington, DC; 2004.

3. Swann AC, Bowden CL, Morris D, Calabrese JR, Petty F, Small J, Dilsaver SC, Davis JM. Depression during mania. Treatment response to lithium or divalproex. *Arch Gen Psychiatry.* 1997; 54(1):37-42.

4. Chan HH, Wing Y, Su R, Van Krevel C, Lee S. A control study of the cutaneous side effects of chronic lithium therapy. *J Affect Disord.* 2000; 57(1-3):107-13.

5. Keck PE, Jr., Strakowski SM, Hawkins JM, Dunayevich E, Tugrul KC, Bennett JA, McElroy SL. A pilot study of rapid lithium administration in the treatment of acute mania. *Bipolar Disord.* 2001; 3(2):68-72.

6. American Psychiatric Association: Practice guideline for the treatment of patients with bipolar disorder (revision). *Am J Psychiatry.* 2002; 159(4 Suppl):1-50.

7. (A.) Isojarvi JI: Reproductive dysfunction in women with epilepsy. *Neurology.* 2003; 61(6 Suppl 2):S27-34(B.) Joffe H. Hall JE, Cohen LS, Taylor AE, Baldessarini RJ. A putative relationship between valproic acid and polycystic ovarian syndrome: implications for treatment of women with seizure and bipolar disorders. *Harv Rev Psychiatry.* 2003; 11(2):99-108. (C.) Meo R. Bilo L. Polycystic ovary syndrome and epilepsy: a review of the evidence. *Drugs.* 2003; 63(12):1185-227.

8. Keck PE, Jr.: The management of acute mania. *British Medical Journal.* 2003; 327(7422):1002-3.

9. Vasudev K, Goswami U, Kohli K. Carbamazepine and valproate monotherapy: feasibility, relative safety and efficacy, and therapeutic drug monitoring in manic disorder. *Psychopharmacology* (Berl). 2000; 150(1):15-23.

10. Moller HJ, Nasrallah HA. Treatment of bipolar disorder. *J Clin Psychiatry.* 2003; 64 Suppl 6:9-17; discussion 28.

11. Simpson GM, Glick ID, Weiden PJ, et. al. Randomized, controlled, double-blind comparison of the efficacy and tolerability of ziprasidone and olanzapine in acutely ill patients with schizophrenia and schizoaffective disorder. *Am J Psychiatry.* 2004; 161: 1837-1847.

12. Hirschfeld RMA, Keck PE, Jr, Kramer M, et. al. Rapid antimanic effect of risperidone monotherapy: a 3-week multicenter, double-blind, placebo-controlled trial. *Am J Psychiatry.* 2004; 161: 1057-1065.

13. Keck PE, Marcus R, Tourkodimitris S, Ali M, Liebeskind A, Saha A, Ingenito G. A placebo-controlled, double-blind study of the efficacy and safety of aripiprazole in patients with acute bipolar mania. *Am J Psychiatry.* 2003; 160: 1651-1658.

14. Turrone P, Kapur S, Seeman MV. Elevation of prolactin levels by atypical antipsychotics. *Am J Psychiatry.* 2002; 159: 133-135.

15. Gupta S, Masand P. Aripiprazole: review of its pharmacology and therapeutic use in psychiatric disorders. *Ann Clin Psychiatry.* 2004; 16: 155-166.

16. Daniel DG. Tolerability of ziprasidone: an expanding perspective. *J Clin Psychiatry.* 2003; 64, Suppl 19, 40-49.

17. Nasrallah HA, Tandon R. Efficacy, safety and tolerability of quetiapine in patients with schizophrenia. *J Clin Psychiatry.* 2002; 63 Suppl 13: 12-20.

18. Conley RR, Meltzer HY. Adverse events related to olanzapine. *J Clin Psychiatry.* 2000; 61 Suppl 8: 26-29.

19. Wirshing DA, Pierre JM, Erhart SM, Boyd JA. Understanding the new and evolving profile of adverse drug effects in schizophrenia. *Psychiatr Clin North Am.* 2003; 26(1):165-90.

20. Barbini B, Scherillo P, Benedetti F, Crespi G, Colombo C, Smeraldi E. Response to clozapine in acute mania is more rapid than that of chlorpromazine. *Int Clin Psychopharmacol.* 1997; 12(2):109-12.

21. Calabrese JR, Kimmel SE, Woyshville MJ, Rapprot DJ, et. al. Clozapine for treatment-refractory mania. *Am J of Psychiatry.* 1996. 153(6): 759-764.

22. Fehr B, Ozcan M, Suppes T. Low Doses of Clozapine may Stabilize Treatment Resistant Bipolar Patients. *Archives of European Psychiatry.* 2004, in press.

23. Keck PE, Jr., McElroy SL. Second generation antipsychotics in the treatment of bipolar disorder. (In Press)

24. Sachs, G, Chengappa KNR, Suppes T, Mullen JA, Brecher M, Devine NA, Sweitzer DE. Quetiapine with lithium or divalproex for the treatment of bipolar mania: a randomized, double-blind, placebo-controlled study. *Bipolar Disorders.* 2004. 6(3):213-224.

25. Muller-Oerlinghausen B, Retzow A, Henn FA, Giedke H, Walden J. Valproate as an adjunct to neuroleptic medication for the treatment of acute episodes of mania: a prospective, randomized, double-blind, placebo-controlled, multicenter study. European Valproate Mania Study Group. *J Clin Psychopharmacol.* 2000; 20(2):195-203.

26. Tohen M, Chengappa KN, Suppes T, Zarate CA, Jr., Calabrese JR, Bowden CL, Sachs GS, Kupfer DJ, Baker RW, Risser RC, Keeter EL, Feldman PD, Tollefson GD, Breier A. Efficacy of olanzapine in combination with valproate or lithium in the treatment of mania in patients partially nonresponsive to valproate or lithium monotherapy. *Arch Gen Psychiatry.* 2002; 59(1):62-9.

27. Freeman MP, Stoll AL. Mood stabilizer combinations: a review of safety and efficacy. *Am J Psychiatry.* 1998; 155(1):12-21.

28. Tohen M, Jacobs TG, Grundy SL, McElroy SL, Banov MC, Janicak PG, Sanger T, Risser R, Zhang F, Toma V, Francis J, Tollefson GD, Breier A. Efficacy of olanzapine in acute bipolar mania: a double-blind, placebo-controlled study. The Olanzipine HGGW Study Group. *Arch Gen Psychiatry.* 2000; 57(9):841-9.

29. Post RM, Uhde TW, Roy-Byrne PP, Joffe RT. Correlates of antimanic response to carbamazepine. *Psychiatry Res.* 1987; 21(1):71-83.

Chapter 9: Antidepressant Agents

Mood stabilizers, some anticonvulsants, atypical antipsychotics, and antidepressant agents are used in the treatment of patients with acute bipolar depression. The primary goal of therapy with these agents is to ameliorate acute depressive symptoms without inducing manic, hypomanic, or mixed symptoms or episodes. This chapter discusses different classes of drugs related to the treatment of bipola depression.

Several different classes of medication have been used to treat symptoms of acute bipolar depression. These include lithium,

Chapter 9 at a Glance

anticonvulsants, atypical antipsychotics (newer generation psychotropics), Selective Serotonin Reuptake Inhibitors (SSRIs), bupropion, venlafaxine, tricyclic antidepressants (TCAs), and Monoamine Oxidase Inhibitors (MAOIs).

The mechanisms of action of these classes of agents differ considerably from each other, even within the same class. While various agents have similar efficacy, each antidepressant drug has its own advantages and disadvantages.

Based on clinical trial results, lithium and the anticonvulsant lamotrigine are recommended by the American Psychiatric Association Guidelines as first-line therapy for acute bipolar depression. Valproate, carbamazepine, and topiramate are other anticonvulsants being studied for the treatment of patients with acute bipolar depression.[1-3] Since publication of these guidelines, the combination of olanzapine and fluoxetine (Symbyax®) was the first formulation to receive a U.S. FDA indication for the acute treatment of bipolar depression for the atypical antipsychotics. Among atypical antipsychotics, randomized, controlled trials in acute bipolar depression have been conducted only with olanzapine, quetiapine, and risperidone.

SSRIs are commonly prescribed antidepressants with efficacy in patients with both unipolar and bipolar depression. They are generally preferred to MAOIs and TCAs because of their tolerability and favorable side effect profile. Of the SSRIs, fluoxetine, paroxetine, and citalopram have been found to be effective for the treatment of acute bipolar depression when combined with a mood stabilizer.[4-6] These medications are often considered first-line treatments due to their favorable side-effect profile. Since the introduction of SSRIs, TCAs (e.g., imipramine, amitriptyline) and other

For dosing, administration, drug interactions, and side effects of lithium, divalproex, carbamazepine, and atypical antipsychotics, see chapter 8.

antidepressants like bupropion or venlafaxine are considered second- or third-line agents, although they may be preferred in individual cases.

Generally, antidepressant treatment is divided into three phases: acute, continuation, and maintenance. Once the decision is made to add an antidepressant to mood stabilizer therapy for a patient with bipolar depression, acute treatment is initiated.

Lithium

Based on clinical trial results over four decades, lithium is recommended as first-line therapy for treatment of acute bipolar depression by the American Psychiatric Association Guidelines (by definition).[1]

For lithium side effects, administration, toxicity and drug interactions, see chapter 8

Clinical Trial Results

Early trials of lithium in the 1960s in patients with acute bipolar depression reported that lithium was superior in efficacy to placebo: 36 percent of patients had an unequivocal response and 79 percent had at least partial benefit.[7] In recent studies patients with lithium levels below 0.8 mEq/L benefited from a combination of lithium and paroxetine. Above these lithium levels, however, there were no added antidepressant benefits from the addition of paroxetine or imipramine in this trial.[8] Thus, other antidepressants may not be required in patients with acute bipolar depression treated with lithium unless the patient cannot tolerate full lithium therapy. Young et. al. conducted a study of combination lithium plus valproate mood stabilizer therapy compared with monotherapy with either drug plus paroxetine.[9] While the two regimens had equivalent efficacy, the combination mood stabilizer regimen was not as well tolerated as monotherapy plus an antidepressant.

Anticonvulsants

Lamotrigine

Lamotrigine, along with lithium, is recommended by the American Psychiatric Association Guidelines as first-line therapy for acute bipolar depression. Lamotrigine is chemically unrelated to existing antiepileptic drugs.[10]

Clinical Trial Results

In a randomized, placebo-controlled, seven-week study of 195 patients with acute bipolar depression, treatment with lamotrigine at 50 mg/d and 200 mg/d was superior to placebo, and switch rates into hypomania or mania did not differ between groups.[10] Subsequently, the efficacy of lamotrigine in acute bipolar depression was confirmed in a parallel-group, flexible dose study and a double-blind crossover trial.[11, 12] However, because lamotrigine appears to have no acute antimanic properties, many patients will also require a mood stabilizer such as lithium.[13]

Pharmacology

Lamotrigine, in part, appears to exert its antiepileptic and antidepressant properties by modulating voltage-sensitive sodium channels and inhibiting the release of excitatory neurotransmitters.[14] Following oral administration, the drug is rapidly absorbed and reaches peak plasma concentrations within 1.4 – 4.8 hours. When taken with meals, absorption is slightly delayed. Lamotrigine is approximately 55 percent bound to plasma proteins. Its volume of distribution is approximately one L/kg. With multiple doses, the drug's elimination half-life is approximately 26.4 hours.

Lamotrigine metabolism occurs predominantly by conjugation with glucuronic acid in the liver; approximately 70 percent is then excreted in the urine. Because metabolic and excretory pathways are hepatic and renal, lamotrigine should be administered cautiously in patients with liver and kidney disease. There are no significant age-related pharmacokinetic issues.

Drug Interactions

In patients also receiving valproate, the lamotrigine dose should be reduced by approximately 50 percent to minimize potential toxicity and decrease risk of potentially serious rash. Valproic acid reduces the clearance of lamotrigine from the plasma and prolongs the drug's elimination half-life. As a result, lamotrigine levels are elevated approximately two-fold.[1]

Anticonvulsant drugs that upregulate hepatic drug-metabolizing activity, such as carbamazepine, increase plasma clearance and reduce lamotrigine's elimination half-life. With carbamazepine, initial starting dose is often doubled, and target dose is higher. Oxcarbazepine does not effect the metabolism of lamotrigine to the same degree as carbamazepine. When combined with oxcarbazepine, initial starting dose should be the one used when no valproate or carbamazepine is used.

Side Effects

Common side effects associated with lamotrigine include:

- Neurologic changes: headache, dizziness, diplopia, ataxia
- Fatigue, asthenia, nausea, dry mouth
- Hypersensitivity reactions
- Cutaneous manifestations,
- Rarely, Stevens-Johnson syndrome (toxic epidermal necrolysis)

Following the recommended medication-dosing schedule is critical because of the risk (rare) of a medically serious rash (Stevens-Johnson syndrome or toxic epidermal necrolysis). This syndrome is strongly associated with absolute starting dose and/or rate of initial titration.

Administration

During the first two weeks, lamotrigine should usually be administered at a dose of 25 mg/d. The dose can then be doubled (50 mg/d) for weeks three and four. Thereafter, the dose can be increased in weekly increments of 50–100 mg/d to a maximum of 200–400 mg/d. To reduce the potential for a hypersensitivity reaction, lamotrigine should **NOT** be titrated upward rapidly. In fact, slow titration appears to reduce the risk of serious rash in lamotrigine-treated patients to that observed with other antiepileptic drugs.[1] To decrease the likelihood of rash development, avoid initiating treatment immediately following a viral syndrome, using new chemicals (e.g., skin products or detergents) within eight weeks after lamotrigine treatment begins, or coming in contact with poison ivy/oak. If discontinuing lamotrigine for any reason for more than five days, it must be re-titrated from a starting dose amount.

Divalproex/Valproate/Valproic Acid

There are no published, controlled trials of valproate or its various formulations in the treatment of acute bipolar depression. Thus, no recommendations can be made with regard to its use for this indication. Chapter 8 includes detailed information on valproate therapy on pages 8-11 through 8-15.

Carbamazepine

The principles behind carbamazepine therapy have been described in chapter 8. For dosage administration, side effects, and drug interactions, see pages 8-15 through 8-18 of that chapter.

Clinical Trial Results

In a small, double-blind, placebo-controlled crossover study, Ballenger et. al. reported that 44 percent of patients with acute bipolar depression experienced a significant improvement from baseline with carbamazepine therapy.[15] In a more recent study, Dilsaver et. al., demonstrated significant improvement in patients with acute bipolar depression treated with carbamazepine.[16] A subset of patients with mixed episodes was less likely to respond to the drug, however.

Topiramate

Topiramate is a sulfamate-substituted monosaccharide. Although originally approved by the FDA for the treatment of partial seizures in adults, it has also been found to be useful in a number of non-seizures disorders. These include bipolar disorder, neuropathic pain, migraine, binge eating, etc.

Pharmacology

While the drug's exact mechanism of action is not totally clear, basic science studies have demonstrated several concentration-dependent properties that appear to contribute to topiramate's overall activity. These include a time-dependent inhibition of neuronal action potentials, potentiation of GABAergic inhibitory activity, and activation of the kainate/AMPA subtype of the glutamatergic receptor. The drug also inhibits carbonic anhydrase. Topiramate is rapidly absorbed from the gastrointestinal tract with peak plasma concentrations occurring approximately two hours after an oral dose. The drug has a bioavailability of approximately 80 percent; availability not affected by food. After single or multiple doses, the mean plasma elimination half-life is 21 hours. Steady state concentrations are reached in four days. Unlike many of the other antiepileptic drugs, topiramate has minimal plasma protein binding (13–17 percent). Approximately 70 percent of topiramate is excreted unchanged in the urine. Since topiramate is significantly excreted into the urine, the dose is usually decreased by approximately 50 percent in patients with moderate or severe renal impairment. In patients with liver disease, topiramate clearance may be reduced by a poorly understood process. Age, gender, and race do not affect the drug's pharmacokinetics.

Drug Interactions

Since topiramate can produce depression of the CNS, it should be used with caution in patients with a history of barbiturate or ethanol abuse. Topiramate alters the pharmacokinetics of combination oral contraceptive pills and metformin. Consequently, contraceptive efficacy can be impaired and diabetic control disrupted in patients taking topiramate and either drug.

Side Effects

The most common adverse effects identified in topiramate-treated subjects are somnolence, fatigue, psychomotor slowing, difficulties concentrating, language problems (e.g., difficulties finding the "correct word"), paresthesias and decreased appetite. Treatment with topiramate has been rarely associated with acute myopia and secondary angle-closure glaucoma.

Administration

For patients with seizures, the recommended dose of topiramate is 400 mg/d, administered in two divided doses. Initiate treatment at a dose of 25–50 mg/d and then titrated in 25–50 mg increments weekly to an effective dose. In most patients, it is unnecessary to monitor plasma drug concentrations. Outpatient dosing may be lower in patients with bipolar disorder.

Topiramate Efficacy

There are no placebo-controlled trials of topiramate in the treatment of acute bipolar depression.[17] However, several trials suggest that it may be effective as an adjunctive measure.[18, 19]

Atypical Antipsychotics (Newer Generation Psychotropics)

Some atypical antipsychotics have been shown to have mood stabilizing properties. Therefore, as a class, they might be anticipated to have efficacy in patients with acute bipolar depression, although at present only the olanzapine-fluoxetine combination is approved by the FDA for the treatment of bipolar depression.

Chapter 8 reviews dosage, administration, and side effects of the newer generation atypical antipsychotics.

Among atypical antipsychotics, randomized, controlled trials in acute bipolar depression (to date) have been conducted only with olanzapine, quetiapine, and risperidone.

Olanzapine

Tohen, et. al. conducted a double-blind, randomized, placebo-controlled, eight-week trial of olanzapine (5–20 mg/d), olanzapine-fluoxetine combination (6 & 25, 6 & 50, 12 & 50 mg/d), versus placebo. At eight weeks, the olanzapine, olanzapine/fluoxetine, and placebo groups demonstrated MADRS total scores lower than baseline by 15.0, 18.5, and 11.9 respectively.[20]

Quetiapine

Calabrese, et. al. presented the results of an eight-week, multicenter, double-blind, randomized, fixed-dose, placebo-controlled trial of quetiapine (300 mg/d, 600 mg/d) monotherapy in outpatients with bipolar I or II disorder (n = 511) with a current episode of depression lasting at least four weeks.[21] At eight weeks, the 300-mg, 600-mg, and placebo groups demonstrated lower than baseline MADRS total score by 16.39 (57 percent reduction), 16.73 (58 percent reduction), and 10.26 (36 percent reduction), respectively. The effect size was .73 for the quetiapine 300 mg/d group and .88 for the 600-mg/d group.[21]

Risperidone

In a small randomized, 12-week trial, Shelton et. al. studied the effects of mood stabilizers in combination with adjunctive risperidone (1–6 mg/d) or paroxetine (20–40 mg/d), with similar doses of risperidone or paroxetine plus placebo, in patients with acute bipolar depression.[22] All three treatment groups showed similar reductions in MADRS scores.

Selective Serotonin Reuptake Inhibitors (SSRIs)

SSRIs are commonly prescribed antidepressants that have efficacy in patients with both unipolar and bipolar depression. They are preferred to MAOIs and TCAs in many situations because of their tolerability and favorable side-effect profile. However, like other antidepressants, the SSRIs must be administered in conjunction with a mood stabilizer to prevent mood switches and cycle acceleration in patients with acute bipolar depression.

Clinical Trial Results

Of the SSRIs, fluoxetine, paroxetine, and citalopram have been studied and found to be effective as add-on therapy for the treatment of acute bipolar depression. The results suggest that patients with acute bipolar depression can be effectively treated with the combination of a mood stabilizer plus an SSRI. It is generally assumed that sertraline and fluvoxamine will show similar results; however, this has not been formally studied in bipolar depression.

In a study of 89 lithium-treated subjects with acute bipolar depression, treatment with fluoxetine produced improvement in 86 percent of patients.[5] This result was not only significantly better than placebo (p=0.005) and the tricyclic antidepressant imipramine (p<0.05), but significantly fewer fluoxetine-treated patients discontinued therapy because of adverse events. It should be noted that using the more modern analyses of in-least-to-treat response rates with fluoxetine decreases the results to about 60 percent, and that some patients were also receiving lithium.

The efficacy and safety of paroxetine add-on therapy was compared with combination lithium and valproate in 27 patients randomized to paroxetine or a second mood stabilizer.[9] While improvements from baseline in Hamilton Depression Scale scores were significant and equivalent for both groups at week 6 (p<0.001), more patients treated with lithium plus valproate dropped out of the trial. A second study confirmed the efficacy of paroxetine in lithium-treated patients, although efficacy over placebo was restricted to those with lithium levels less than 0.8 mEq/L.[4]

In an open, add-on treatment study of patients with bipolar I and II, citalopram has also been reported to have efficacy in this indication.[6]

A recent search of *Medline* and related sources found no trials using sertraline or fluvoxamine. However, in clinical practice, sertraline is often one of the SSRIs of choice for bipolar depression treatment.[23]

Pharmacology

Although the exact mechanism of action of SSRIs in depression is still somewhat unclear, several effects appear to contribute to the activity of the class, including:

1. Inhibition of neuronal reuptake of serotonin from the synaptic cleft

2. Desensitization of serotonergic feedback receptors

3. Downregulation of β-adrenergic receptors

Since clinical efficacy is often not seen for four to six weeks, the selective serotonin reuptake inhibition that occurs within hours is not solely responsible for the efficacy effect.

SSRIs are administered orally and well absorbed from the gastrointestinal tract. Their half-life varies from 15 to 20 hours (fluvoxamine) up to 7 to 10 days (fluoxetine plus its active metabolites).[14] While the drug's elimination half-life does not affect efficacy or onset of action, it is an important consideration when the dose must be altered due to side effects or drug-drug interactions.

Side Effects

SSRI side effects relate to their effects on various neurotransmitters and receptors (see table 9-1 on page 9-13).

Key considerations related to these side effects include:

• Adverse events in the GI tract are due to a combination of the drug's muscarinic and histaminergic blockade and activation of serotonergic receptors.

- Neurologic manifestations are secondary to blockade of the muscarinic and histaminergic receptors plus stimulation of the noradrenergic, serotonergic, and dopaminergic receptors.

- Cardiovascular side effects result from alpha1-adrenergic blockade and activation of noradrenergic and dopaminergic receptors.

Drug Interactions

SSRIs are metabolized by hepatic cytochromes, principally CYP2D6 and CYP3A3/4. Consequently, there is the potential for drug interactions when they are co-administered with drugs that act as competitive inhibitors or inducers of various cytochromes. The prescribing information for each individual drug should be examined for potential side effects before an SSRI is prescribed.

Table 9-1. SSRI Side Effects in Relation to Their Effects on Neurotransmitter and Receptor Activity

Location of Side Effect	Symptoms	Receptor Activity
Gastro-intestinal	Dry mouth, constipation	Muscarinic blockade
	Weight gain	Histaminergic blockade
	Loss of appetite, nausea, vomiting, diarrhea	Serotonergic stimulation
Neurological	Blurred vision	Muscarinic blockade
	Sedation	Histaminergic blockade
	Anxiety, insomnia, tremor, diaphoresis	Noradrenergic stimulation
	Sexual dysfunction, akathisia, headache, insomnia	Serotonergic stimulation
	Agitation, psychosis	Dopaminergic stimulation
Cardio-vascular	Orthostatic hypotension	Alpha-1 adrenergic blockade
	Elevated blood pressure	Dopaminergic or noradrenergic stimulation
	Tachycardia	Noradrenergic stimulation

Contraindications

Agents of this class should not be combined with MAOIs because of the risk of the serotonergic syndrome: confusion, tremor, myoclonus, hypertension, hyperthermia, and diarrhea. Hypericum perforatum, also known as St. John's Wort, is an herbal preparation with natural antidepressant properties sold in extract form in health food stores. Because of the drug's non-selective blockade of serotonergic, noradrenergic, and dopaminergic receptors, significant side effects such as the serotonergic syndrome can occur when patients are also receiving antidepressant therapy. In an attempt to manage depressive symptoms, some patients may self-medicate with this herb.

Other Antidepressants

Before the SSRIs and other alternative antidepressants were introduced, a tricyclic antidepressant (TCA) was the add-on drug of choice for the treatment of acute bipolar depression. However, TCAs are now generally considered second- or third-line agents for this indication.

Tricyclic Antidepressants

Clinical Trial Results

In general, treatment of acute bipolar depression with a TCA results in response rates that are superior to placebo and equivalent to or somewhat less effective than the comparators.[1] However, treatment with these drugs is accompanied by a higher rate of manic or hypomanic switch than other antidepressants. For example, in the study conducted by Nemeroff et. al. of lithium plus paroxetine, six to 11 percent of patients treated with imipramine had a treatment-induced switch compared with only two and zero percent in the placebo and paroxetine-treated subjects, respectively.[4]

Pharmacology

Members of the TCA family share a chemical structure that contains at least two, joined benzene rings.[14]

Side Effects

Side effects result from the activity of the drugs as blockers of various receptors: muscarinic, histaminergic, and adrenergic. In general, TCAs that are secondary amines are less likely to produce anticholinergic and histaminergic adverse events.

Contraindications

The various TCAs are classified as class I antiarrhythmic drugs. TCAs should often be avoided in patients with a history of heart disease and in individuals treated with other drugs that can impair cardiac conduction (e.g., quinidine, procainamide) because their activity on cardiac sodium

> *TCAs should be prescribed with caution to patients with acute bipolar depression who are also suicidal. An overdose of even one week's worth of medication is potentially fatal.*

channels leads to a decrease in impulse propagation through the cardiac conduction system. Consequently, they can produce QTc prolongation, left bundle branch block, complete heart block, and/or sudden death.

Bupropion

Pharmacology

Bupropion is an aminoketone antidepressant chemically unrelated to other agents of this class. Although its exact mechanism of action is not precisely known, bupropion inhibits the neuronal uptake of both dopamine and norepinephrine. Experimentally, the drug acts as a stimulant and can cause seizures in large doses. The drug is rapidly absorbed following administration, metabolized and activated in the liver, and excreted in the urine.

Side Effects

Key considerations related to bupropion side effects include:

- Immediate-release bupropion in doses up to 450 mg/d induces seizures in approximately 0.4 percent (4/1000) patients.

- The incidence of seizures in patients treated with extended-release bupropion is similar to that reported with SSRI treatment. The risk of seizures increases at doses over 450 mg/d in patients with epilepsy, bulimia nervosa, and head trauma. Bupropion levels can be elevated when co-administered with agents that interfere with its metabolism.

- Bupropion can produce agitation, insomnia, delusions, hallucinations, and weight loss.

- Bupropion induces hepatic cytochromes, and its metabolism can be affected by other drugs processed by the CYP450 system.

- Bupropion is generally safe for patients with cardiac disease.

- Bupropion is not significantly associated with the side effects of sexual dysfunction associated with SSRIs.

Drug Interactions

Bupropion induces hepatic cytochromes and can have its metabolism modified by other drugs processed by elements of the CYP450 system. The drug is generally safe in patients with cardiac disease and is not associated with the sexual dysfunction produced by the SSRIs. In patients with acute bipolar depression maintained on mood modifiers, treatment with bupropion was as effective as desipramine and less likely to precipitate a manic episode than the TCA (11 percent versus 30 percent).[24]

Venlafaxine

Clinical Trial Results

In a study of venlafaxine and paroxetine in 60 women with acute bipolar depression treated with mood stabilizers, 48 percent of the patients treated with venlafaxine had a 50 percent or greater decrease in baseline Hamilton depression scores (p<0.0001).[25] Although efficacy was equivalent to that produced by the SSRI, more patients treated with venlafaxine (13 percent versus three percent) had a switch to hypomania or mania.

Pharmacology

Venlafaxine is a phenethylamine bicyclic drug chemically unrelated to other antidepressants. It appears to potentiate CNS neurotransmitter activity through serotonin/norepinephrine reuptake inhibition. The drug is also a weak inhibitor of dopamine reuptake. Venlafaxine is rapidly absorbed following oral administration, metabolized in the liver by CYP2D6, and excreted in the urine. Consequently, its pharmacokinetic properties are extensively modified by the presence of hepatic and/or renal disease.

Side Effects

Side effects of venlafaxine include those typical of SSRIs and a risk of hypertension at higher doses.

Monoamine Oxidase Inhibitors (MAOIs)

Clinical Trial Results

MAOIs increase the concentration of monoamines at the synapse and appear to be superior to TCAs in their antidepressant activity in bipolar depression. Studies of the MAOI tranylcypromine demonstrated that it was more effective than imipramine. For example, compared with imipramine, patients with acute bipolar depression treated with tranylcypromine had significantly greater symptomatic improvement and global response rates as well as lower attrition rates than those who received the TCA.[20] The risk for developing mania is high when used without antimanic agents.[1, 7] Because of safety issues, this group of medications are considered second- or third-line choices for treatment of bipolar depression.

Pharmacology

Monoamine oxidase (MAO) catalyzes the oxidative degradation of monoamines such as dopamine, serotonin, norepinephrine, and tyrosine. In the liver, MAO catabolizes monoamines from the gastrointestinal tract that are absorbed into the portal circulation.

Side Effects

Side effects, which are due to inhibition of MAO activity, include postural hypotension, sexual dysfunction, insomnia, weight changes, and peripheral neuropathy, which can often be prevented by the prophylactic administration of pyridoxine (vitamin B_6).

Toxicity

Inhibition of MAO in the liver is responsible for the systemic toxicity that can be observed with this class of drug. For example, patients treated with foods rich in monoamines can experience an adrenergic crisis that results in hypertension, tachycardia, arrhythmias, hyperpyrexia, and tremulousness. Hypertension in patients with severe adrenergic reactions can cause intracranial hemorrhage. The classic example of an adrenergic crisis occurs when a patient treated with an MAOI attends a wine- and cheese-tasting party and becomes severely symptomatic after tasting red wine and strong or aged cheeses.

References

1. American Psychiatric Association: Practice guideline for the treatment of patients with bipolar disorder (revision). *Am J Psychiatry.* 2002; 159(4 Suppl):1-50.

2. Post RM, Uhde TW, Roy-Byrae PP, et. al. Antidepressant effects of carbomazepine. *Am J Psychiatry.* 1986; 43: 29-34.

3. Small JG. Anticonvulsants in affective disorders. *Psychopharmacology Bulletin.* 1990; 26: 25-76.

4. Nemeroff CB, Evans DL, Gyulai L, Sachs GS, Bowden CL, Gergel IP, Oakes R, Pitts CD. Double-blind, placebo-controlled comparison of imipramine and paroxetine in the treatment of bipolar depression. *Am J Psychiatry.* 2001; 158(6):906-12.

5. Cohn JB, Collins G, Ashbrook E, Wernicke JF. A comparison of fluoxetine imipramine and placebo in patients with bipolar depressive disorder. *Int Clin Psychopharmacol.* 1989; 4(4):313-22.

6. Kupfer DJ, Chengappa KN, Gelenberg AJ, Hirschfeld RM, Goldberg JF, Sachs GS, Grochocinski VJ, Houck PR, Kolar AB. Citalopram as adjunctive therapy in bipolar depression. *J Clin Psychiatry.* 2001; 62(12):985-90.

7. Zornberg GL, Pope HG, Jr. Treatment of depression in bipolar disorder: new directions for research. *J Clin Psychopharmacol.* 1993, 13(6).397-408.

8. Nemeroff CB, Evans DL, Gyulai L, Sachs GS, Bowden CL, Gergel IP, Oakes R, Pitts CD. Double-blind, placebo-controlled comparison of imipramiine and paroxetine in the treatment of bipolar depression. *Am J Psychiatry.* 2001; 158(6):906-12.

9. Young LT, Joffe RT, Robb JC, MacQueen GM, Marriott M, Patelis-Siotis I. Double-blind comparison of addition of a second mood stabilizer versus an antidepressant to an initial mood stabilizer for treatment of patients with bipolar depression. *Am J Psychiatry.* 2000; 157(1):124-6.

10. Calabrese JR, Bowden CL, Sachs GS, Ascher JA, Monaghan E, Rudd GD. A double-blind placebo-controlled study of lamotrigine monotherapy in outpatients with bipolar I depression. Lamictal 602 Study Group. *J Clin Psychiatry.* 1999; 60(2):79-88.

11. Bowden CL. Novel treatments for bipolar disorder. *Expert Opin Investig Drugs.* 2001; 10(4):661-71.

12. Frye MA, Ketter TA, Kimbrell TA, Dunn RT, Speer AM, Osuch EA, Luckenbaugh DA, Cora-Ocatelli G, Leverich GS, Post RM. A placebo-controlled study of lamotrigine and gabapentin monotherapy in refractory mood disorders. *J Clin Psychopharmacol.* 2000; 20(6):607-14.

13. Keck PE, JR., McElroy SL. Treatment of bipolar disorder. *Textbook of Psychopharmacology,* 3rd Edition. Nemeroff CB, Schatzberg AF, eds. American Psychiatric Publishing, Inc., Washington, DC, 2004.

14. Goodman LS, Hardman JG, Limbird LE, Gilman AG. *Goodman & Gilman's the pharmacological basis of therapeutics.* New York: McGraw-Hill; 2001.

15. Ballenger JC, Post RM. Carbamazepine in manic-depressive illness: a new treatment. *Am J Psychiatry*. 1980; 137(7):782-90.

16. Dilsaver SC, Swann SC, Chen YW, Shoaib A, Joe B, Krajewski KJ, Gruber N, Tsai Y. Treatment of bipolar depression with carbamazepine: results of an open study. *Biol Psychiatry*. 1996; 40(9):935-7.

17. Suppes T. Review of the use of topiramate for treatment of bipolar disorders. *JClin Psychopharmacol*. 2002. 22 (6): 599-609.

18. McIntyre RS, Mancini DA, McCann S, Srinivasan J, Sagman D, Kennedy SH. Topiramate versus bupropion SR when added to mood stabilizer therapy for the depressive phase of bipolar disorder: a preliminary single-blind study. *Bipolar Disord*. 2002; 4(3):207-13.

19. Hussein M. Treatment of bipolar depression with topiramate (abstract). *Eur Neuropsychopharmacol*. 1999; 9 (Suppl):S222.

20. Tohen M, Vieta E, Calabrese J, Keter TA, Sachs G, Bowden C, Mitchell PB, Centorrino F, Risser R, Baker RW, Evans AR, Beymer K, Dube S,Tollefson GD, Breier A. Efficacy of olanzapine and olanzapine-fluoxetine combination int he treatment of bipolar I depression. *Archives of General Psychiatry*. 2003b: 60: 1079-88.

21. Calabrese JR, Keck PE, MacFadden W, Minkurtz M, Ketter TA, Weisler RH, Cutler AJ, McCoy R, Wilson E, Mullen J, for the BOLDER Study Group. A randomized, double blind, placebo-controlled trial of quetiapine in the treatment of bipolar I or II depression. *Am J Psychiatry*. 2004, in press.

22. Shelton RC, Addington S, Augenstein E, Ball W. Risperidone and paroxetine in bipolar disorder., in *American Psychiatric Association Annual Meeting*. New Orleans, LA, 2001.

23. Gyulai I, Bowden CL, McElroy SL, Calabrese JR, Petty F, Swann AC, Chou JC, Wassef A, Risch CS, Hirschfeld RM, Nemeroff CB, Keck PE Jr., Evans DL, Wozniak PJ. Maintenance efficacy of divalproex in the prevention of bipolar depression. *Neuropsychopharmacology*. 2003. 28(7): 1374-82.

24. Sachs GS, Lafer B, Stoll AL, Banov M, Thibault AB, Tohen M, Rosenbaum JF. A double-blind trial of bupropion versus desipramine for bipolar depression. *J Clin Psychiatry*. 1994; 55(9):391-3.

25. Vieta E, Martinez-Aran A, Goikolea JM, Torrent C, Colom F, Benabarre A, Reinares M. A randomized trial comparing paroxetine and venlafaxine in the treatment of bipolar depressed patients taking mood stabilizers. *J Clin Psychiatry*. 2002; 63(6):508-12.

26. Himmelhoch JM, Thase ME, Mallinger AG, Houck P. Tranylcypromine versus imipramine in anergic bipolar depression. *Am J Psychiatry*. 1991; 148(7):910-6.

Chapter 10: Maintenance Treatment Options

One of the most important long-term goals of therapy in patients with bipolar disorder is to prevent the recurrence of additional mood episodes. Since approximately 90 percent of patients who experience a manic episode will have recurrent episodes, it is important not only to treat the initial manic/hypomanic or major depressive episode but also to prevent subclinical or clinical relapses.[1] Maintenance therapy is intended to achieve this objective.

Mood stabilizer therapy is the mainstay of maintenance therapy for patients with bipolar disorder. While monotherapy would be ideal, in practice many patients require more than one medication for long term mood stabilization. The efficacy of lithium, lamotrigine, and olanzapine in relapse prevention in bipolar I disorder has been demonstrated in placebo-controlled, long-term trials. Valproate, carbamazepine, clozapine, and aripiprazole also appear to have efficacy in the maintenance treatment of bipolar disorder in controlled trials. Patients treated with a mood stabilizer plus an atypical antipsychotic

---

Chapter 10 at a Glance

---

also appear to have a lower risk of relapse if the combination is continued as maintenance treatment.

When selecting specific maintenance therapy for patients with bipolar disorder, important considerations include:

- Severity of disease
- Presence of rapid cycling and/or psychosis
- Reasonable patient preferences
- Co-occurring medical or psychiatric illnesses

Mood Stabilizers

As mood stabilizers recommended for maintenance therapy, lithium has robust evidence and valproic acid formulations also has demonstrated efficacy.[2] Lamotrigine, an antiepileptic drug, also has mood stabilizing properties. The combination of lithium for prevention of mania and lamotrigine for depression control may be particularly valuable, although this has not yet been demonstrated in a randomized, controlled trial.

Lithium

Clinical Trial Results

Lithium is the best-studied and established agent for the maintenance therapy of patients with bipolar disorder. Placebo-controlled, randomized studies conducted in the 1960s to 1970s demonstrated that maintenance therapy with lithium provides a four-fold advantage compared with placebo for preventing relapse at 6- and 12-month intervals.[3] See the section on page 10-4 covering lamotrigine for a description of recent 18-month, placebo-controlled trials.

Response Factors

When considering lithium maintenance therapy, it is important to consider factors that may reduce response to the drug.[4] (See table 10-1 on the next page.)

Table 10-1. Factors that Impair Response to Lithium Maintenance Therapy[4]

◆ Rapid cycling

◆ Multiple prior mood episodes

◆ Absence of a family history of mood disorders

◆ Associated alcohol or substance use disorder

◆ Episode sequence of depression-mania-euthymia

From Bowden CL. Predictors of response to divalproex and lithium. *J Clin Psychiatr.* 1995;56(Suppl):25-30.

Maintaining Optimal Serum Lithium Levels

To maximize outcomes of lithium maintenance therapy, serum lithium levels usually need to be maintained at a level of 0.6–0.8 mEq/L or higher.[5] Several studies have demonstrated that lithium levels in the 0.4 mEq/L to 0.6 mEq/L range are associated with relapse rates and subsyndromal manifestations that are 2.6-fold greater than those seen in patients with levels of 0.8 mEq/L or greater.[6, 7] Importantly, however, higher lithium levels are associated with greater toxicity and associated discontinuations. Therefore, the optimal serum lithium level in an individual patient is one that achieves the best efficacy tolerability ratio.

Chapter 8 (pages 8-6 through 8-8) describes lithium side effects in detail.

Anticonvulsants – Clinical Trial Results

Valproate

Bowden et. al. found that divalproex-treated patients (compared with the placebo controlled group), had lower rates of discontinuation for either a recurrent mood episode or depressive episode.[8]

Two open-label studies compared valproate with lithium as maintenance therapy in patients with bipolar disorder. In one study, both drugs had comparable efficacy, while in the other,

> *Chapter 8 (pages 8-12 through 8-13) describes valproate side effects in detail.*

the relapse rate of patients treated with the valpromide formulation of valproate was 20 percent lower than that of lithium after 18 months.[9, 10]

Lamotrigine

Two studies with similar designs evaluated the efficacy and tolerability of lamotrigine plus lithium for the prevention of mood episodes/relapses in outpatients with bipolar disorder over 18

> *Chapter 9 (page 9-5) describes lamotrigine side effects in detail.*

months.[11, 12] Both lamotrigine and lithium were superior to placebo at prolonging the time to intervention for any mood episode. Lamotrigine

was statistically superior to placebo at prolonging the time to intervention for a depressive episode, while lithium was statistically superior to placebo at prolonging the time to intervention for a manic or hypomanic episode.

Carbamazepine

Due to methodological issues, the results of most studies of carbamazepine for the maintenance therapy of patients with bipolar disorder are often difficult to interpret. Two recent studies compared the drug with lithium. In the first study, relapse rates for carbamazepine and lithium did not significantly differ after one year (37 percent versus 31 percent, respectively).[13]

> *Chapter 8 (pages 8-16 through 8-17) describes carbamazepine side effects in detail.*

However, results obtained in the trial's third year indicated that the combination of lithium and carbamazepine was superior to monotherapy with either drug.

In the second trial, however, carbamazepine was inferior to lithium at 2.5 years in a number of outcome measures; however, carbamazepine provided a superior benefit to patients with atypical symptoms.[14]

At this time, no study evidence exists on the relationship between serum carbamazepine levels and response rates.

Atypical Antipsychotics (Newer Generation Psychotropics) – Clinical Trial Results

Atypical antipsychotics provide a favorable risk-benefit profile in the treatment of acute bipolar disorder relative to the older typical antipsychotics. They are particularly useful when the episode is severe or when it is accompanied by psychotic manifestations. Evolving evidence suggests that these agents may have a role in long-term therapy of patients with bipolar disorder.

The clinical trial results described for the following medications represent completed controlled maintenance or prophylactic trials. We can anticipate an increase in information in this area as a number of controlled trials are underway.

Clozapine

Suppes et. al. studied the efficacy of long-term clozapine in 38 patients with treatment-resistant schizoaffective or bipolar disorder in a randomized, open-label study.[15] Patients were randomized to clozapine add-on or treatment as usual (no clozapine) and followed for one year. There were significant between-group differences on all clinical symptom scales except for depression. Patients with bipolar I disorder without psychotic symptoms who received clozapine showed improvement similar to that of the entire clozapine-treated group and required lower doses than those with schizoaffective illness.

Olanzapine

Based on clinical trial evidence, olanzapine has recently been approved by the U.S. FDA for maintenance therapy of bipolar disorder. One trial found that olanzapine-treated patients had significantly lower rates of manic relapse compared with lithium-treated patients.[16] Other research found patients on olanzapine had less manic and depressive recurrence than the placebo group, and that olanzapine performed as well as divalproex in rates of mania remission.[17, 18]

Aripiprazole

Keck et. al. studied the long-term efficacy of aripiprazole in 161 bipolar I patients with a recent manic or mixed episode.[19] Patients who had been stabilized on aripiprazole were randomized to placebo or aripiprazole for a 26-week maintenance phase. Aripiprazole significantly prolonged time to relapse in bipolar

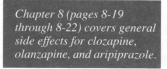
Chapter 8 (pages 8-19 through 8-22) covers general side effects for clozapine, olanzapine, and aripiprazole.

I patients, most recent episode manic or mixed. The number of relapses to any type episode was also significantly lower in the aripiprazole group.

Managing Patients Who Fail to Respond

Lithium and lamotrigine efficacy for preventing recurrent manic and depressive episodes, respectively, suggests that it is reasonable to consider this combination. Similarly, the combination of olanzapine with lithium or divalproex was superior to lithium or divalproex alone in relapse prevention.[20]

When patients continue to experience breakthrough symptoms or mood instability, the clinician should first ensure that drug levels are within the therapeutic range. If levels are in the low- to mid-range and side effects are minimal, increase maintenance dosing to achieve a level at the higher end of the therapeutic range.

For patients who fail to respond to this approach, mood stabilizers may be supplemented with a second maintenance agent, such as one of the following:

- Lamotrigine
- Another antiepileptic drug
- An atypical antipsychotic
- An antidepressant

At this time, data are insufficient to make a more definitive recommendation. The updated Texas Medication Algorithms (expected publication in 2005) will address currently available maintenance data and provide general recommendations.

References

1. Hopkins HS, Gelenberg AJ. Treatment of bipolar disorder: how far have we come? *Psychopharmacol Bull.* 1994; 30(1):27-38.

2. Keck PE, Jr., McElroy SL: Treatment of bipolar disorder. *American Psychiatric Association Textbook of Pschopharmocology*, 3ʳᵈ ed. APPI. Washington, DC; 2004.

3. Keck PE, Jr., Welge JA, Strakowski SM, Arnold LM, McElroy SL. Placebo effect in randomized, controlled maintenance studies of patients with bipolar disorder. *Biol Psychiatry.* 2000; 47(8):756-61.

4. Bowden CL. Predictors of response to divalproex and lithium. *J Clin Psychiatry.* 1995; 56(Suppl):25-30.

5. Baldessarini RJ, Tondo L, Hennen J, Viguera AC. Is lithium still worth using? An update of selected recent research. *Harv Rev Psychiatry.* 2002; 10(2):59-75.

6. Gelenberg AJ, Kane JM, Keller MB, Lavori P, Rosenbaum JF, Cole K, Lavelle J. Comparison of standard and low serum levels of lithium for maintenance treatment of bipolar disorder. *N Engl J Med.* 1989; 321(22):1489-93.

7. Keller MB, Lavori PW, Kane JM, Gelenberg AJ, Rosenbaum JF, Walzer EA, Baker LA. Subsyndromal symptoms in bipolar disorder. A comparison of standard and low serum levels of lithium. *Arch Gen Psychiatry.* 1992; 49(5):371-6.

8. Bowden CL, Calabrese JR, McElroy SL, Gyulai L, Wassef A, Petty F, Pope HG, Jr., Chou JC, Keck PE, Jr., Rhodes LJ, Swann AC, Hirschfeld RM, Wozniak PJ. A randomized, placebo-controlled 12-month trial of divalproex and lithium in treatment of outpatients with bipolar I disorder. Divalproex Maintenance Study Group. *Arch Gen Psychiatry.* 2000; 57(5):481-9.

9. Revicki D, Hirschfeld R, Keck PJ. Cost-effectiveness of divalproex sodium vs. lithium in long-term therapy for bipolar disorder., in *American College of Neuropsychopharmacology Annual Meeting.* San Juan, PR. 1999.

10. Lambert P, Vernaud G. Comparative study of valpromide versus lithium as prophylactic treatment of affective disorders. *Nervure J Psychiatrie.* 1982; 4:1-9.

11. Bowden CL, Calabrese JR, Sachs G, Yatham LN, Asghar SA, Hompland M, Montgomery P, Earl N, Smoot TM, DeVeaugh-Geiss J. A placebo-controlled 18-month trial of lamotrigine and lithium maintenance treatment in recently manic or hypomanic patients with bipolar I disorder. *Arch Gen Psychiatry.* 2003; 60(4):392-400.

12. Calabrese JR, Bowden CL, Sachs G, Yatham LN, Behnke K, Mehtonen OP, Montgomery P, Ascher J, Paska W, Earl N, DeVeaugh-Geiss J. A placebo-controlled 18-month trial of lamotrigine and lithium maintenance treatment in recently depressed patients with bipolar I disorder. *J Clin Psychiatry.* 2003; 64(9):1013-24.

13. Denicoff KD, Smith-Jackson EE, Disney ER, Ali SO, Leverich GS, Post RM. Comparative prophylactic efficacy of lithium, carbamazepine, and the combination in bipolar disorder. *J Clin Psychiatry*. 1997; 58(11):470-8.

14. Greil W, Ludwig-Mayerhofer W, Erazo N, Schochlin C, Schmidt S, Engel RR, Czernik A, Giedke H, Muller-Oerlinghausen B, Osterheider M, Rudolf GA, Sauer H, Tegeler J, Wetterling T. Lithium versus carbamazepine in the maintenance treatment of bipolar disorders--a randomised study. *J Affect Disord*. 1997; 43(2):151-61.

15. Suppes T, Webb A, Paul B, Carmody T, Kraemer H, Rush AJ. Clinical outcome in a randomized 1-year trial of clozapine versus treatment as usual for patients with treatment-resistant illness and a history of mania. *Am J Psychiatry*. 1999; 156(8):1164-9.

16. Tohen M, Marneros A, Bowden C, et.al. Olanzapine versus lithium in relapse prevention in bipolar disorder: a randomized double-blind controlled 12-week trial. *Abstracts of the New Clinical Drug Evaluation Unit Annual Meeting*. May 26-28, 2003, Boca Raton, FL.

17. Tohen M, Ketter TA, Zarate CA, Suppes T, Frye M, Altshuler L, Zajecka J, Schuh LM, Risser RC, Brown E, Baker RW. Olanzapine versus divalproex sodium for the treatment of acute mania and maintenance of remission: a 47-week study. *Am J Psychiatry*. 2003; 160(7):1263-71.

18. Tohen B, Bowden C, Calabrese J, et. al. Olanzapine's efficacy for relapse prevention in bipolar disorder: a placebo-controlled, randomized, double-blind controlled 12-month trial. *Abstracts of the Fifth International Conference on Bipolar Disorder*. June 16, 2003, Pittsburgh, PA.

19. Keck PE, Sanchez R, Marcus RN, Carson WH, Rollin L, Iwamoto T, Stock EG. Aripiprazole for relapse prevention in bipolar disorder in a 26-week trial. *Presented at The 157th Meeting of the American Psychiatric Association*. May 1 6, 2004a; New York, NY.

20. Tohen M, Chengappa KN, Suppes T, Baker RW, Zarate CA, Bowden CL, Sachs GS, Kupfer DJ, Ghaemi SN, Feldman PD, Risser RC, Evans AR, Calabrese JR. Relapse prevention in bipolar I disorder: 18-month comparison of olanzapine plus mood stabiliser v. mood stabiliser alone. *Br J Psychiatry*. 2004. 184:337-45.

Chapter 11: Psychosocial Interventions for Bipolar Disorder

While psychosocial interventions were once the only available option for patients with bipolar disorder, they now comprise an important adjunctive treatment to psychopharmacology. Psychosocial therapies can help patients and their families understand the disease, adhere to medications, manage stress, and prevent relapse.

Table 11-1, on page 11-3, summarizes the four main types of psychosocial interventions: psychoeducation, problem solving/coping, family-focused treatment, and psychotherapy.

Psychoeducational Interventions

The patient and family should be educated about the nature of bipolar illness. Disease-state education can be introduced early during treatment and become more detailed as the patient progresses in therapy, emphasizing education about the disorder managing stress, and preventing relapse.

Education about the disorder addresses the:

- Lifelong nature of the disorder
- Prodromal symptoms
- Treatment benefits

Chapter 11 at a Glance

- Rationale behind drug therapy and potential side effects
- Importance of adherence to therapy
- Skills for dealing with common illness issues
- Communication strategies with physicians

Stress management psychoeducation stresses:

- That stress can precipitate new mood episodes
- How to obtain support resources
- Techniques for organizing daily activities into a regular pattern, which reduces stress in various domains

Relapse prevention psychoeducation stresses:

- How to avoid environmental factors that may precipitate a relapse
- Potential indicators of recurrent disease
- The value of a regular sleep/wake schedule

Problem–Solving/Coping Interventions and Family-Focused Treatment (FFT)

Problem-solving/coping interventions and Family-focused Treatment (FFT) predominately assist the patient in navigating through work problems, resolving family issues, and reaching life's goals. Family-focused treatment (FFT) is based on the assumption that environment determines a component of the patient's risk of relapse. FFT includes:

1. **Psychoeducation** — about the disorder and how it effects the family

2. **Communication Enhancement Training** — to reduce stressful interpersonal relationships

3. **Problem-solving Skills Training** — to identify, define, and solve specific, bipolar illness-related problems in the family setting

Table 11-1. Psychosocial Interventions

Type	Objectives	Potential Strategies
Psychoeducational Interventions	• Teach patient and family members about the nature of the disorder and bipolar disorder management skills • Provide reading materials and videos supporting these topics	• Stressing importance of medication adherence • Promoting medication compliance • Identifying potential precipitating factors • Recognizing early relapse
Problem Solving/Coping Interventions	• Help the patient function in various domains (e.g., social, work, financial) • Help the patient identify and attain life goals	• Discussing problem-solving techniques in various domains (e.g., negotiating with supervisors at work, marital issues) • Identifying realistic life goals (e.g., completing education, seeking employment, leisure-time activities)
Family-Focused Treatment Interventions	• Assist the patient with resolving interpersonal issues that may result from the illness or associated psychiatric comorbidities	• Participating in family or marital therapy to improve communications and problem solving between family members
Psychotherapeutic (IPSRT and CBT) Interventions	• Help the patient accept loss • Build the patient's self-image and confidence • Focus on maintaining stable life habits and managing stress	• Identifying and reducing feelings of sadness or grief resulting from loss of a loved one, a job, personal possessions, or inability to meet unrealistic goals • Helping the patient achieve a healthy, realistic self-image • Helping patients establish consistent eating and sleeping schedules

Psychotherapy (Interpersonal and Cognitive Behavioral)

In **Interpersonal and Social Rhythm Therapy (IPSRT),** patients learn to monitor the relationships between their mood and daily routines, sleep, and interactions with others to develop insights into the interdependence of the various domains. Patients learn to anticipate and address events that can disrupt their normal routines and potentially precipitate mood episodes.

Cognitive Behavioral Therapy (CBT) is a technique to help patients modify their thinking and reactions to various life situations, including self-perceptions, their psychiatric disorder, and disease-associated problems.[1] Patients who are educated about their illness are better prepared to participate in their treatment and maintenance phases by defining realistic goals and monitoring progress toward achieving these goals.

Efficacy of Psychosocial Interventions for Bipolar Mood Presentations

Although more randomized clinical trials are needed, accumulating evidence indicates that psychosocial interventions are feasible and can contribute to improved outcomes in patients with bipolar disorder.[2] Table 11-2, on the following pages, presents an overview of key research conducted on Psychoeducation, FFT, IPSRT, and CBT.

Table 11-2. Psychosocial Intervention Efficacy

Type of Intervention	Comparator	Nature of Subjects Studied	Key Results
Psycho-education (21 structured group sessions)	Matched, randomized group of non-structured group meetings[3]	• N=120 • Patients received standard pharmaco-therapy	• Psychoeducation group experienced: — Significantly reduced recurrences — Increased time between episodes — Decreased number and length of hospitalizations
Family-Focused Therapy (FFT)	Two, family education sessions and crisis management[4]	• N=101 • Patients also received pharmaco-therapy	• FFT: — Decreased relapse rate after 1 year (29% vs. 53%)* — More effective in preventing depression relapse — Resulted in less severe depressive symptoms
	Individually focused therapy[5]	• N= 53 • Patients also received pharmaco-therapy	• FFT decreased: — Relapse rate (28% vs. 60%)* — Hospitalization (12% vs. 60%)*
	Two, family education sessions with crisis management[6]	• N=101 • Patients also received pharmaco-therapy	• FFT: — Decreased relapse rate (35% vs. 54%)* — Increased relapse-free interval (73.5 vs. 53.2 weeks)* — Improved medication adherence

* (First % is FFT; second % is comparator)

Table 11-2 continued

Type of Intervention	Comparator	Nature of Subjects Studied	Key Results
Inter-personal and Social Rhythm Therapy (IPSRT)	Intensive clinical management[7, 8]	• Large maintenance trial • Patients also received pharmaco-therapy	• IPSRT increased stability of daily routines and sleep/wake cycles. • Patients treated with IPSRT for at least 1 year were more likely to remain euthymic. • Consistency of intervention (1 regimen or the other) was associated with lower rates of relapse (20% vs. 40%) over 1 year.**
	Weekly psychosocial therapy over 6 months[9]	• N = 65 • Study of thyroid function with secondary endpoint of response to antide-pressants • Patients also received pharmaco-therapy	• IPSRT failed to produce an additive benefit on relief of depressive symptoms or time to remission.

** Patients were re-randomized during the study. Those randomized to continue in the same group had improved outcomes.

Table 11-2 continued

Type of Intervention	Comparator	Nature of Subjects Studied	Key Results
Cognitive Behavioral Therapy (CBT)	Pharmacotherapy alone (Lithium)[10]	• Intervention group received pharmacotherapy plus 6 weeks of CBT	• CBT: —Improved medication adherence —Decreased mood disorder hospitalizations during 6 months of follow up
	Routine care including pharmacotherapy[11]	• N=69 • Patients also received pharmacotherapy	• CBT resulted in: — Self-identification of early mood symptoms and earlier medical intervention —30% reduction in manic relapses —Significantly improved social functioning over 18 months
	Routine care including pharmacotherapy[12]	• N=42 • Patients also received pharmacotherapy	• CBT significantly: —Reduced depressive symptoms —Improved global functioning —Reduced relapse rates in those who switched to CBT after 6 months (60% reduction) compared to routine care alone
	Pharmacotherapy with mood stabilizer[13]	• N = 11 • Patients also received pharmacotherapy	• The addition of CBT to mood stabilizer pharmacotherapy was as effective as CBT alone for patients with unipolar depression.

References

1. Basco MR, Rush AJ. *Cognitive-Behavioral Therapy for Bipolar Disorder.* Guilford Press; New York, 1996.

2. Patelis-Siotis I, Young LT, Robb JC, Marriott M, Bieling PJ, Cox LC, Joffe RT. Group cognitive behavioral therapy for bipolar disorder: a feasibility and effectiveness study. *J Affect Disord.* 2001; 65(2):145-53.

3. Colom F, Vieta E, Martinez-Aran A, Reinares M, Goikolea JM, Benabarre A, Torrent C, Comes M, Corbella B, Parramon G, Corominas J. A randomized trial on the efficacy of group psychoeducation in the prophylaxis of recurrences in bipolar patients whose disease is in remission. *Arch Gen Psychiatry.* 2003; 60(4):402-7.

4. Miklowitz DJ, Simoneau TL, George EL, Richards JA, Kalbag A, Sachs-Ericsson N, Suddath R. Family-focused treatment of bipolar disorder: 1-year effects of a psychoeducational program in conjunction with pharmacotherapy. *Biol Psychiatry.* 2000; 48(6):582-92.

5. Rea MM, Tompson MC, Miklowitz DJ, Goldstein MJ, Hwang S, Mintz J. Family-focused treatment versus individual treatment for bipolar disorder: results of a randomized clinical trial. *J Consult Clin Psychol.* 2003; 71(3):482-92.

6. Miklowitz DJ, George EL, Richards JA, Simoneau TL, Suddath RL. A randomized study of family-focused psychoeducation and pharmacotherapy in the outpatient management of bipolar disorder. *Arch Gen Psychiatry.* 2003; 60(9):904-12.

7. Frank E, Swartz HA, Kupfer DJ. Interpersonal and social rhythm therapy: managing the chaos of bipolar disorder. *Biol Psychiatry.* 2000; 48(6):593-604.

8. Frank E, Swartz HA, Mallinger AG, Thase ME, Weaver EV, Kupfer DJ. Adjunctive psychotherapy for bipolar disorder: effects of changing treatment modality. *J Abnorm Psychol.* 1999; 108(4):579-87.

9. Cole DP, Thase ME, Mallinger AG, Soares JC, Luther JF, Kupfer DJ, Frank E. Slower treatment response in bipolar depression predicted by lower pretreatment thyroid function. *Am J Psychiatry.* 2002; 159(1):116-21.

10. Cochran SD. Preventing medical noncompliance in the outpatient treatment of bipolar affective disorders. *J Consult Clin Psychol.* 1984; 52(5):873-8.

11. Perry A, Tarrier N, Morriss R, McCarthy E, Limb K. Randomised controlled trial of efficacy of teaching patients with bipolar disorder to identify early symptoms of relapse and obtain treatment. *Bmj.* 1999; 318(7177):149-53.

12. Scott J, Garland A, Moorhead S. A pilot study of cognitive therapy in bipolar disorders. *Psychol Med.* 2001; 31(3):459-67.

13. Zaretsky AE, Segal ZV, Gemar M. Cognitive therapy for bipolar depression: a pilot study. *Can J Psychiatry.* 1999; 44(5):491-4.

Index

Trisha Suppes, M.D., Ph.D.
Statement of Disclosure

Sources of Funding for Clinical Grants: Dr. Suppes is a principal or co-investigator on research studies sponsored by Abbott Laboratories, AstraZeneca Pharmaceuticals, Bristol Meyers Squibb, Glaxo Smith Kline Pharmaceuticals, Janssen Pharmaceutica, National Institutes of Mental Health, Novartis, Robert Wood Johnson Pharmaceutical Research Institute, and The Stanley Medical Research Institute.

Consulting Agreements/Advisory Boards/Speaking Bureaus: Dr. Suppes is a consultant to, or member of the scientific advisory boards of Abbott Laboratories, AstraZeneca Pharmaceuticals, Bristol Meyers Squibb, Eli Lilly Research Laboratories, Glaxo Smith Kline Pharmaceuticals, Janssen Pharmaceutica, Johnson & Johnson Pharmaceutical Research & Development, Novartis Pharmaceutical, Pfizer, Pharmaceutical Research Institute (PRI), Ortho McNeil Pharmaceutical, Shire Pharmaceutical, Solvay Pharmaceutical, and UCB Pharma.

Paul F. Keck, Jr. M.D.
Statement of Disclosure

Research Grants: Dr. Keck is a principal or co-investigator on research studies sponsored by Abbott Laboratories, the American Diabetes Association, AstraZeneca, Bristol-Myers Squibb, GlaxoSmithKline, Elan, Eli Lilly, Janssen Pharmaceutica, Merck, National Institute of Mental Health (NIMH), National Institute of Drug Abuse (NIDA), Organon, Ortho-McNeil, Pfizer, the Stanley Medical Research Institute (SMRI), and UCB Pharma.

Consultant/Scientific Advisory Boards: Dr. Keck is a consultant to, or member of the scientific advisory boards of Abbott Laboratories, AstraZeneca Pharmaceuticals, Bristol-Myers Squibb, GlaxoSmithKline, Janssen Pharmceutica, Jazz Pharmaceuticals, Eli Lilly and Company, Novartis, Ortho-McNeil, Pfizer, UCB Pharma, Shire, and Wyeth.

Compact Clinicals Publications

For Physicians

Bipolar Disorder: Treatment and Management
By Trisha Suppes, MD, PhD & Paul E. Keck, Jr., MD

For Clinicians

Aggressive and Defiant Behavior
The Latest Assessment and Treatment Strategies for the Conduct Disorders
By J. Mark Eddy, PhD

Attention Deficit Hyperactivity Disorder
The Latest Assessment and Treatment Strategies
By Keith Conners, PhD

Bipolar Disorder
The Latest Assessment and Treatment Strategies
By Trisha Suppes MD, PhD and Ellen Dennehy, PhD

Borderline Personality Disorder
The Latest Assessment and Treatment Strategies
By Melanie Dean, PhD

Depression in Adults
The Latest Assessment and Treatment Strategies
By Anton Tolman, PhD

Obsessive Compulsive Disorder
The Latest Assessment and Treatment Strategies
By Gail Steketee, PhD and Teresa Pigot, MD

Post Traumatic Stress Disorder
The Latest Assessment and Treatment Strategies
By Mathew J. Friedman, MD, PhD

For more information or to order, contact:
Compact Clinicals
7205 N.W. Waukomis Drive
Kansas City, MO 64151
1-800-408-8830